HOW TO REDUCE YOUR CHRONIC PAIN:

A New Model to Help You Restore Hope

By
Dr. George Beilin
Licensed Psychologist

Wendy & Paul
I do hope you
find the way to reduce pain
over time helpful!
Stay resilient! [illegible]

Published by Dr. Painless Publishing

ISBN 978-0-9996198-0-3
First edition: 2018

Editor: Kate Victory Hannisian, Blue Pencil Consulting
Book and Cover Design: Brian Murphy Art and Design
Printing: King Printing Co., Inc.

This book is
dedicated to the millions
of people who suffer
with chronic pain daily
and to those people
who care for them.

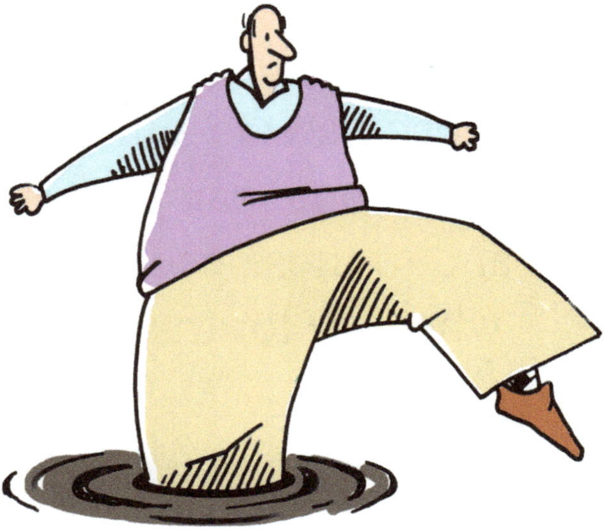

Taking the first step out of the swamp is the hardest.

Contents

Foreword

Thank goodness, the urgent need for a truthsayer has been answered in this wonderfully thoughtful book by Dr. George Beilin. Patients suffering from chronic pain will benefit from the book's ample wisdom, a powerful salve with the potential to help them experience enriched living.

Chronic pain is not only an increasingly pervasive medical condition, as Dr. Beilin explains, but also one that is uniquely challenging for healthcare professionals and their patients, and the family members who support them. The pain can be intractable with persistent, continuous or intermittent debilitating symptoms. It's hard to define and to target with effective, economical and safe treatments. Chronic pain is exceedingly complex because it is so multifaceted and not entirely predictable. Ambiguous working definitions and the limitations of language and speech to express and communicate the human experience of pain complicate the situation. Relying exclusively on drug-based interventions can create dependencies on substances like opioids, which can become addictive and even lethal. We see a crisis today because that trend has now reached epidemic proportions. There's a real need for a safer way to manage chronic pain.

We humans are sensitive creatures who pride ourselves on being intelligent life forms. Yet pain touches the deepest and most fundamental spiritual, philosophical and religious ways of understanding that bind our families and societies together in pursuit of progress. Because these traditions are not entirely consistent or sometimes even compatible, their notions of human behavior and motivation are sometimes hard to reconcile. No wonder healers can seem so inconsistent or unenlightening to patients in dire need of immediate answers. That same obstacle is exasperating and frustrates the very self-confidence and motivation that patients need in order to sustain their recovery efforts. The disappointments and delays also trigger reactions that deplete the perseverance and good intentions of supporting family and friends, and Dr. Beilin teaches us that this can also interfere with progress or even set back the best efforts of all involved.

Indeed, chronic pain is a quagmire with contradictions and competing agendas and priorities at every turn. For Heaven's sake, what can one do to avoid hopeless despair, frivolous expenditures of energy and precious finances, and instead actually produce genuine healing and resolution?

Fortunately, Dr. George Beilin contributes something that is comprehensive in its scope, heartfelt, readily understandable, and remarkably likely to be effective. In my long career as a healthcare provider and an attorney, I have experienced many people with serious medical and physical conditions, as well as emotional and psychological ones. These people experience excruciating distress both from the pain and the stressors of modern life. I have been working for several decades in teaching hospitals (such as Massachusetts General Hospital/Harvard Medical School and Tufts Medical School), public agencies and state facilities, the military, and at Harvard Law School. As a clinician, teacher, and supervisor, I can certainly attest that my colleague Dr. Beilin is one of the most outstanding and brilliant professionals I have encountered, and he well deserves my highest respect and regard for his understanding, compassion, expertise, skill, ethics and empathetic concern. It is my pleasure to encourage you to read carefully and follow the sound advice he has laid out so elegantly and sensibly in this book.

Dr. Beilin has drawn upon and blended resources from Western and Eastern cultural traditions in order to create a comprehensive and effective coping stratagem to help us handle life's most compelling challenges, including chronic pain.

What I appreciate most is his offering of methodical exercises and approaches you can use to improve your life experience in the face of many different challenges, most notably those you face if you have chronic pain. Dr. Beilin's new model does a superior job of distinguishing adaptive from maladaptive strategies for pain management and boosting motivation necessary to achieve, sustain, and renew the motivation that's essential for change. His model is also based on standard empirical assessment and monitoring procedures to more reliably detect, measure and document actual experiential results.

What I find most impressive in George's model is his incorporation of the most recent and powerful understanding in the field of psychology regarding choice and free will. The eminent Israeli psychologist Daniel Kahneman, author of *Thinking, Fast and Slow,* won a Nobel Prize for the ground-breaking research that he and my graduate school classmate Amos Tversky conducted in behavioral economics theory. They studied how people really make choices, considering that humans are not entirely rational, but instead subject to profound cognitive biases and heuristic thinking. In this book, Dr. Beilin superbly explains in layman's terms this remarkably important refinement of Freudian notions about dynamic unconscious that have prevailed for the past century. The genius in these insights is that cognitive appraisal becomes a tool that chronic pain patients can use to reduce the panoply of types of "*pain*." Dr. Beilin correctly explains that painful experiences are really not simply medical phenomena, but are instead an amalgam of physical, emotional, life stressor and other factors.

Dr. George Beilin's insights are truly the fruition and culmination of both the Western cultural tradition's pathways for understanding human nature and the Eastern tradition's contributions of meditational mindfulness. "*Positive Psychology*," à la Dr. Martin Seligman, a former president of the American Psychological Association, is a cornerstone of Dr. Beilin's methodology, which has distilled and translated the pivotal aspects of time-honored and tested wisdom for coping. Dr. Beilin's book brings contemporary insights about human nature and societal organization to key ideas from the third century BC in a form that reflects the Age of Reason and modern science.

Best wishes on your journey using Dr. Beilin's model for a Pain Management Lifestyle. You have suffered enough and no longer need to be saddled with the disabling and debilitating pain that has been torturing you. It is time to take control and seize the opportunity to live life fully and unencumbered by misery.

Steven Nisenbaum, PhD, JD
Medical Staff, Psychiatry Department,
Massachusetts General Hospital/School of Medicine
Assistant Clinical Professor in Public Health and Community Medicine,
Tufts Medical School

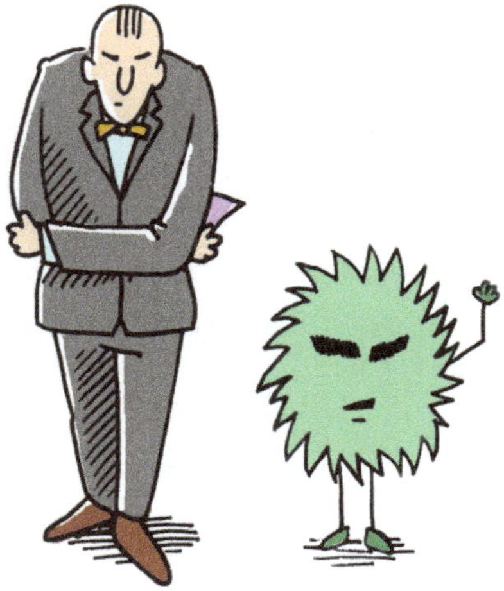

Let's welcome Chronic Pain! Right here! On our stage!

INTRODUCTION

"Pain is inevitable; suffering is optional."
M. Kathleen Casey

Yes, you have chronic pain. Don't let anyone tell you differently. While others try to minimize it, the pain continues to exist. It has been with you for well over three months. It may be sharp, stinging, or a dull ache. It may be a tingling sensation in your fingers and toes or a feeling of stiffness or heaviness, or an achy feeling that seems to come and go with no rhyme or reason. You want to scream in agony, pray for relief, cry from constant suffering as you lie there in bed covered by a blanket, or while sitting up or walking even short distances.

Others around you who don't have chronic pain just don't seem to understand. They try to comfort and reassure you, but it just doesn't do any good. The pain just eats away at your inner core. They tell you to "Live with it!", "Be strong!" or "Ignore it!" It seems so easy for them to say these things when you still have the torturing pain. You become more irritable, angry and hypersensitive to everything they say. You think, ***"Oh, it's so easy to give suggestions!"*** Meanwhile, the pain increases even when you do what your doctor or clinical nurse practitioner tells you to do. You take medications that do nothing for the pain. You know the medical community is cutting back on prescribing certain painkillers because they're worried about drug abuse. The pain comes right back to haunt you. You agonize about the future; you worry that the pain will only get worse; you fear that it will always be like this and it will never get better no matter what you try.

You think about what you did to deserve this suffering. You feel such guilt for anything you might have said or done over the years and for what others around you have had to endure since feeling the pain. You apologize continuously to others and to G-d; yet the pain still eats away at you and you don't know why. You generate constant, anxious and depressing thoughts. Your life stress is unbearable. The pain is so intense that at times you feel like it's not worth living, that you simply want to die. You withdraw in your bed, hoping that the next day will bring you some relief. But it doesn't.

You are not alone if you've experienced any of these thoughts or feelings. In fact, there are presently about 100 million people in the United States who suffer from chronic pain. That's approximately 1 in every 3.5 people. About 25 million of them describe their pain as being moderate to severe in intensity. Approximately 2 out of 3 people in pain have had it for more than five years "Chronic pain costs the nation up to $635 billion each year in medical treatment and lost productivity," according to a study released in 2011 ("Relieving Pain in America: A Blueprint for Transforming Prevention, Care, Education, and Research," Institute of Medicine Committee on Advancing Pain Research, Care, and Education). The study's authors noted that these expenditures related to pain are higher than those for cancer, heart disease, and diabetes combined. And that's just the physical pain. But what about pain from anxiety, depression, anger or unhappiness? What about pain from negative thinking, life stressors, or from a lack of fortitude?

In this book, you will learn how to reduce all your pain by developing a *"pain management lifestyle."* You will learn ten different facts about pain and about how to use five easy scales that will help you lower your pain levels on a weekly basis. Finally, you will learn specific strategies to use with each scale to reduce and maintain low pain levels over time. If you're ready to learn more about developing your new *"pain management lifestyle,"* read on.

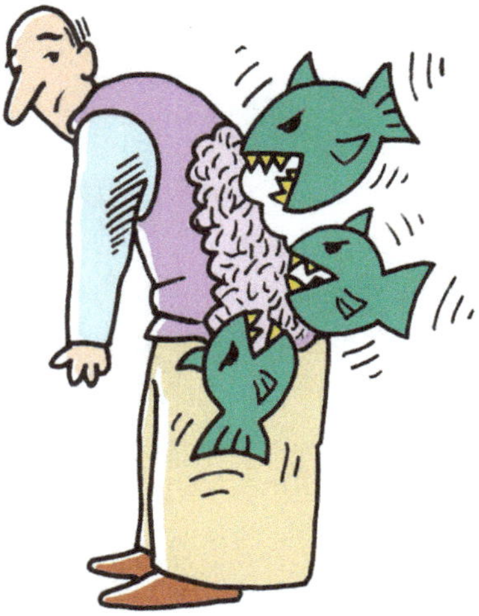

This gnawing pain is too much for me to bear!

Chapter 1: My Story

Everyone who has endured chronic pain has a story to tell – and that includes me. My story began in autumn 2005. Since my late teens, I had been quite an athlete, jogging and playing tennis two to three times a week, biking three to four hours on weekends, climbing mountains and skiing single and double black diamond trails during the winter months. In the early 1980s, I trained for and ran three Boston Marathons, staying in the "back of the pack" just for the thrill of it rather than for speed. I recall having some knee pain after the second marathon in 1981 and went to see orthopedic surgeon Kenneth Greg, who said to me, "George, given your husky size, I'd highly recommend that you run on soft, wooded trails rather than paved roads!" While I felt thin at 185 pounds and 6 feet, I still knew what Dr. Greg meant. Instead of sticking to wooded trails, I rationalized that the endorphin high of street jogging on the sloped, hard pavement would be much nicer. Did I listen to him? No. Who did in those days?

As a licensed psychologist, I did a lot of psychological testing during those years. I typed hundreds of reports, never paying any attention to my own hunched-over posture at my desk. My report writing helped me sustain a large referral base of doctors and nurses, but it never occurred to me what I was doing to my spine. My wife would scold me for bending over forward, pressing down hard on the keyboard with two fingers. I didn't listen to her, just like I didn't listen to Dr. Greg. My frenetic need to get these reports done surpassed any long-term concern for what could happen to my spine and peripheral nerves.

I continued to play tennis often and remained active athletically until 2005 when, at age 54, I noticed some tingling sensations in my fingers and toes. My physician at the time did a blood and urine test and ruled out diabetes. He then referred me to a neurologist who initially observed that my symptoms were probably due to "wearing tight sneakers, and you may have carpal tunnel syndrome." After he administered an Electromyogram (EMG) he told me, "You have peripheral neuropathy." He was an older gentleman and didn't recommend anything for me to do, other than inform me that my peripheral nerve fiber endings were damaged. There was no empathy from him.

I knew I had to stop playing tennis. This was perhaps the most painful experience I confronted at the time. Tennis had been in my blood since childhood. I grew up with a father who became a handball champion in New York City's Bronx neighborhood. He had met my mother while playing mixed doubles with her on a handball court. My parents eventually picked up racket sports and encouraged me to do the same. I recall the thrill of having a wooden Davis racket at age 10 and a natural ability to play singles. Even though my parents couldn't afford to give me tennis lessons or have me train or do United States Tennis Association competitions, I still enjoyed both the competition and the socialization tennis provided. I enjoyed playing at our local tennis courts in Cunningham and Alley Pond Park in Queens in between my elementary school yard stickball games. On weekdays, I often rode my bike to the park after school. I took a bag lunch on weekends and played tennis all day while socializing with other players of all ages who loved the sport.

As a young adult, I remember one spring day playing against a young New York Knickerbocker rookie named Phil "Shoulders" Jackson. Boy, was that fun, as this guy laughed at himself, not knowing how to get out of his own way at the net if I hit a ball directly at him. Every year, I went with some friends to the US Open at the original Forest Hills Stadium off Queens Boulevard. Later on, I would teach tennis lessons at summer camps and continue to play for fun at Ohio State University, then Cunningham and Alley Pond Parks again when I transferred to New York University. After obtaining my bachelor's degree in psychology, I headed for Boston to attend graduate school and played at local park tennis courts in Brookline and Cambridge. Eventually, I obtained my doctoral degree, then married a beautiful woman I met while doing a clinical internship on Boston's North Shore. Stephanie had similar clinical interests and loved athletics as much as I did. We moved to the North

Shore after I obtained my first job as a clinical director of a state Department of Mental Health regional adolescent day program and continued to play in the early mornings at a local club for many years. Tennis was so much a part of me that I envisioned I would eventually die on a tennis court in my later years.

How did your chronic pain begin? Was it a long time in the making or did it come on suddenly through an accident or an illness? What did it force you to give up? How have you mourned it and, more importantly, moved on?

I mourned tennis for a long time after having to give it up. Periodically, I would cry alone in my car while passing the tennis club on my way to the office. I missed the early-bird group of men and women I had come to know since the early 1980s. Yes, I would always have my memories, but it wasn't the same. Grieving anything or anyone that has been a part of your life for so long is tough, no matter what. This is what happens when you begin to have chronic pain.

I eventually had to give up jogging as well because of the ongoing tingling sensations in my feet. Oh boy! A double whammy. To go out jogging at any time was a natural high. Ask any jogger how enjoyable it is to run for miles. One becomes entranced in an endorphin-producing, meditative state after a mile. Not being able to do this ever again made me quite sad, especially when I recalled how I loved jogging with my wife Stephanie, friends or in the woods with one of our golden retrievers.

After letting go of tennis and jogging, I managed to cope by biking during the warm months and by doing the aerobic-elliptical machine at the local YMCA during the winter. Still, it wasn't the same. Losing both the ability to play tennis and jog symbolically represented my entry into a painful rite of passage, namely aging.

Fortunately, I remained resilient enough to compromise with my body. I continued to bike industriously, played golf with my friend on Friday mornings and even swam from time to time at the local YMCA, trying to keep in shape. These activities kept me going despite experiencing increased peripheral neuropathy and some sacroiliac pain.

In late August 2008, my wife and I spent a lovely weekend with my sister-in-law and her boyfriend in the White Mountains in Jackson, New Hampshire. We enjoyed their company, taking time to sit in the cold mountain river, walking the wooded paths and playing golf. We left to go home around three that Sunday afternoon but decided to stop briefly at some outlets in North

Conway, New Hampshire. My wife went shopping while I chose to hang out at the Brookstone store. I didn't mind because I saw that they had some massage chairs ranging in price from $1,500 to $4,900 and I thought that trying one out would be a nice, relaxing way to end our stay in the area. Of course, I wasn't going to buy one. I just wanted to try it out, at my own risk.

I chose to sit in the most expensive, leather-covered massage chair because it had so many options and was quite comfortable. I read the indemnification sheet, with language similar to what you see when skiing the more difficult, triple-diamond trails: "Skiing down this trail can cause death. Go at your own risk!" Clearly, I would not hold the store owners or makers of the machine responsible for my decision to try out the chair. I sat down and turned the chair dial to "Shiatsu massage, moderate intensity." I relaxed and felt these hard steel balls start to roll from the top of my neck down my thoracic and lumbar spine, then down both my legs. It was quite comfortable and enjoyable, so much so that I decided to do it again after the first ten-minute massage. Only this time, I chose to lie down flat on my back and turned up the dial to "Shiatsu, high intensity."

No sooner than the machine started did I became paralyzed -- not physically, but psychologically. I could not move from the lowered seat. Nothing was keeping me there physically. I certainly wasn't buckled in. It was if I had become so startled by this strange, electrical sensation in my neck, then in my upper and lower spine, then legs as the steel balls rotated intensely, that I couldn't move. I'd never felt such an eerie, electrical sensation in all my life.

The massage machine stopped after about 15 minutes. I stood up slowly from the chair and felt this intense tightening of my entire body, as if a cobra was squeezing the life out of me. I couldn't move. I became frightened and broke out in a cold sweat. Eventually, I was able to walk slowly outside and waited patiently for my wife. She soon arrived carrying a few packages, then saw that I was having difficulty walking.

Tears came to my eyes, but I tried to be upbeat, joking that my presumed, temporary paralysis must be some muscle tightness from using the machine. Little did I know that this tension would remain with me for four months.

What professionals did you see once you discovered you had chronic pain? How were they helpful or not helpful? What made you decide to accept some of their recommendations while rejecting others? Who was there to support you through your ordeal, and how were they supportive?

"You'll be fine!" my primary care physician (PCP) said as I put my clothes back on after the exam. "All you have to do is stretch and I think yoga would be very helpful for you." Now this was the guy who had recently won an award for being one of the best physicians on the North Shore. Didn't he realize that I had spent days, even weeks, trying to walk at least 50 feet in the park? My worried wife saw what I was going through and became more concerned than ever about my health. She advocated as much as she could, but it fell on deaf ears. She'd yell at me, "Why don't you change doctors? He's doing nothing for you!" She was right, but I had been with him for years, ever since our kids were young and we belonged to the same havurah (a Jewish alternative religious group).

My physician eventually sent me to see an in-network physiatrist (a physician that specializes in musculoskeletal structure), but he was useless since he recommended nothing other than walking and stretching, just like my PCP. For a while longer, I tried to walk with my wife in the shopping mall or at a local park, but I preferred to sit or lie down after a few steps. The gripping pain radiated through my arms and chest then down my legs. Taking showers was as difficult as getting dressed. Each night, after seeing patients, I came home and immediately hopped into bed. I found that lying flat was the only way to gain some relief from the muscle tightness and excruciating chest and leg pain.

In late October 2008, my wife became visibly upset and spoke to my PCP, telling him l that I couldn't walk, even button a shirt, and that I was getting really depressed. He then ordered a brain MRI after my wife feared that I might have developed a brain tumor. My bank branch manager even saw me walking in the bank once and asked me if I had MS, a condition her husband had at the time. I told her that I had no idea but I hoped that the upcoming brain MRI showed something. Well, it didn't. The MRI was perfectly normal. My wife and I became more puzzled and afraid.

In late November 2008, we had had enough. We decided to demand that my PCP refer me to see a neurologist at Massachusetts General Hospital (MGH). It was clear that yoga and stretching didn't change anything and I was still lucky to walk even 10 feet without experiencing gripping pain that radiated through my chest and arms and down both legs. I had so much difficulty getting in and out of the shower, let alone dressing without assistance. Something had to change.

When we arrived at the MGH Neurology Department early one December morning, the reception staff informed us that we had made an excellent choice in seeing Dr. Gilmore O'Neal, a visiting neurologist and researcher from Ireland. "Thank G-d! Something was going right," I thought. We didn't wait long until a handsome young man dressed in a warm blue suit appeared from behind the reception station and called out, in a clear Irish brogue, "Dr. Beilin?" I got up and slowly walked to meet Dr. O'Neal, who watched me walk then guided me into his office. Dr. O'Neal told me that he noticed how slowly and awkwardly I had walked and that I dragged my feet. I agreed, telling him, "It's been a very difficult few months and very trying on my wife!" (She was as scared as I was.) He then proceeded to ask me for a detailed history, writing intently as I talked about my initial experience with peripheral neuropathy leading to what I considered a traumatic event at the Brookstone store in late August.

Then, he asked me to come into his examining room and change into a johnny, then let him know when I was ready. This didn't take long although I couldn't tie the string of the hospital gown behind my neck. Dr. O'Neal performed a standard neurological examination and inquired where I felt the most pain. I told him, "all over but definitely more in my middle chest and stomach area." Dr. O'Neal said that he wanted me to have a full MRI of my cervical, thoracic and lumbar spine as soon as possible. When I asked what he thought was going on, Dr. O'Neal remained silent, then softly stated that he "still wasn't sure," but that his request for a full MRI "was prudent." Dr. O'Neal had his secretary instruct the Mass General MRI Center in Charlestown to arrange for a full MRI with contrast and secured an opening for the following week.

I'll never forget that cold, raw Friday morning. It had been pouring all night before and continued after I got up at 4 AM to get dressed and headed to Charlestown for a 6 AM appointment. It took about 40 minutes to get there. The heavy rain, intermixed with ice, pounded on my car windshield as I crossed the Tobin Bridge and followed the looping directions past the USS *Constitution* in Charlestown to the MRI Center garage. The MRI scan took approximately 45 minutes. Then I was injected with a dye that would create contrasting images that would help the doctor detect any potential tumors. The technician rolled me back into the machine for an additional 15 minutes for the scan with contrast.

The entire procedure went smoothly. I never had any anxieties about MRIs even with their loud, banging noise. I closed my eyes this time and imagined myself as a young boy, holding my father's hand, watching construction for the lower sections of a new skyscraper being built in Manhattan. I imagined a cluster of people looking through scattered wall openings, watching bulldozers and dump trucks move about like Tonka toys. Like many New Yorkers, I found the repetitious clatter of heavy metal rather meditational.

After I re-dressed, the medical assistant asked me if I wanted to meet the radiologist reviewing my MRI scan. "Of course!" I said. Why wait for a report when I could review the radiologist's opinion immediately? After all, I had some familiarity seeing MRIs of the spine. The medical assistant walked me into a dark room behind multiple machines showing multiple MRI scans. In front of them sat the radiologist, who told me he had already observed my scans but hadn't written the report yet. "Would you like to see them?" he asked. "Absolutely!" I said. He brought up a series of scans, with the first one showing my lumbar spine highlighted in orange. "This is your L4-L5 area. The color indicates that you have severe stenosis at the L4-L5 level." (Stenosis is a narrowing of the vertebrae against the spinal canal.)

"So that's why I have had such pain!" I said, almost relieved to have a physical cause be the answer. But the radiologist said, "No! While this condition is giving you pain, there's another area that you should see!" My throat went dry as the radiologist brought up on the screen a scan of my cervical area. It was bright red. On the scan, one of the cervical vertebrae penetrated one third of the way into my spinal cord. I felt faint.

Being Grateful

Being grateful for the people in your life and the things you already have is a major virtue in helping reduce chronic pain. Martin Seligman, author of *Learned Optimism* (1998) and *Authentic Happiness* (2002) and the founder of the American Psychological Association's Division on Positive Psychology, maintains that expressing gratitude regularly for people or things in your life increases your happiness.

To whom are you grateful for when trying to cope with your chronic pain? What is it about them that made you grateful? What things in your life are you grateful for?

It has been years since I first lay down on that massage chair in the Brookstone store. I am forever grateful to even share my story, given that I thought I was going to die of suffocation by a "neurological boa constrictor" that day. Besides being grateful for eventually meeting Dr. O'Neal, the neurologist at Massachusetts General Hospital, I am forever grateful to Dr. Terrance Doorly, the neurosurgeon who first performed an emergency cervical laminectomy (the removal of a vertebrae lamina) in late December 2008, then two subsequent partial hemilaminotomies (the cleaning out of nerve roots emanating from the spinal cord to peripheral nerves, through the vertebrae) in April 2009 and September 2013. In between, he performed a spinal fusion with instrumentation at L4-L5, in December 2012.

I truly believe that G-d had a major influence in my connecting to this dedicated, spiritual surgeon. Dr. Doorly was one of only two neurosurgeons on the North Shore, but I did have the opportunity to get another reputable neurosurgeon in Boston at Massachusetts General Hospital after I spoke with Dr. O'Neal, who reviewed my MRI report and firmly advised me to "find someone quickly" to perform an emergency cervical laminectomy. He said that he would give me some names of MGH colleagues if I couldn't come up with anyone soon. We were heading into the Christmas and New Year's holidays, when many neurosurgeons wouldn't be available. It turned out that Dr. Doorly was going back to Ireland with his family for a vacation but could perform the surgery just before they left. Many professionals, including my PCP, regarded him highly, as did present and former patients. (Dr. Doorly later came to be affiliated with Massachusetts General Hospital when Partners Healthcare expanded to the North Shore and took over North Shore Medical Center.)

I had become more religious since my father died in 2006, and after my wife and I toured Israel in August 2007. While I attend an Orthodox Temple, I am not an Orthodox Jew. It's just that the traditional prayers and hymns and Torah (the first five books of the Bible) readings remind me so much of the same experiences I recalled growing up in New York.

When I met Dr. Doorly for the first time, I couldn't help but feel positive about being with him. Between meeting Dr. O'Neal and Dr. Doorly, I felt so happy and hopeful enough to dance the Irish jig (with a little Hora interlude, being Jewish). Dr. Doorly had a contagious smile, spoke in a melodious Irish brogue and bounced around his office while talking to his staff in some humorous way. When I first visited him that cold mid-December day, we talked about Ireland and his upcoming visit. He then examined me, observed that I had weak mobility and strength, and had a dropped foot. He then looked closely at the cervical MRI, sighed and stated, "Yup. This one's going to hurt!" That meant he would enter surgically through the deep muscular layer behind my neck. Dr. Doorly went on to not only perform a successful surgery on my cervical spine but three more surgeries to which he could have objected for whatever reason. Since then, I've had two hip replacements (in February 2014 and 2016). That's six surgeries in seven years. I became a "bionic person!"

What strategies did you pursue to help cope with your pain? How were they helpful or not helpful in reducing or not reducing your chronic pain?

Between surgeries, I underwent several physical therapies while continuing to see patients, sometimes until nine at night. I went to two pain management centers after my physical pain increased. I saw one anesthesiologist-pain management physician who recommended and administered multiple cortisone injections. When those procedures provided no symptom relief, that same doctor recommended the insertion of a subcutaneous transdermal nerve stimulator implant (TENS device) underneath my skin. I rejected that recommendation. I learned that there are many people with chronic pain who find such devices helpful in addition to other pain management strategies. I had used an external TENS device and found it helpful to some degree, although I had to be careful about getting skin irritations from where the electrodes were placed.

I became familiar with the internal TENS devices after I made chronic pain management a specialty following my first neurosurgery, then becoming chief psychologist for five years at one pain management center where I saw many patients referred for the psychological evaluation required by insurance prior to surgical insertion of a TENS device. I followed many patients who had the TENS unit inserted. A majority of them found between 20-35% relief. Some complained of the procedure being arduous since anesthesiologists had to redo the placements of wire mesh or reconnect loose electrodes. Others complained that the internal battery had to be recharged frequently or that they felt embarrassed about their appearance.

I saw an anesthesiologist at a different pain management center who, shockingly to me, recommended methadone. After rejecting his advice, I agreed to have him administer a radio frequency ablation procedure where the anesthesiologist burns certain nerves in specific areas to reduce pain sensation. While this procedure can provide relief for some, it didn't do anything for me. I continued to see their clinical nurse practitioner, who told me that I had "failed back surgeries" and that one way to treat me was with opiates. She stated I had "to learn to live with the pain" while proceeding to prescribe me a Buprenorphine (Suboxone) patch, then Percocet. I knew opiate dependence would increase and that this form of pain management would not be the be-all-end-all for pain relief. I weaned myself off the medications in a few months.

After a dismal, painful summer in 2015, I decided to have another lumbar spine MRI. While I was initially discouraged by the radiology report, I did not see the actual MRI. As fate would have it, I learned from a friend about possibly getting an opinion from the Chief of Orthopedic Surgery at Massachusetts General and Newton-Wellesley Hospitals, Dr. Leon Jenis. Initially, he rejected seeing me after reviewing my records (but not the recent MRI), stating he could do nothing further surgically for me. I still wanted to see him, even for a consult, to which he finally agreed. Dr. Jenis and his medical assistant spent about an hour with my wife and me, reviewing my history and looking at my most recent lumbar spine MRI. In a positive tone, he said, "George, all of Dr. Doorly's surgeries were successful. The recent MRI shows no major structural abnormalities that impede your spinal cord. Whatever pain you are still experiencing is related to something we see in many patients who've had multiple surgeries but sit much in between them. You have severe muscle atrophy. What you need to do is exercise more! That includes muscle strengthening and improving your mobility."

My wife and I were elated. Immediately, I canceled all further appointments with the pain management nurse, then eventually joined a great local athletic club after recovering from my last hip replacement surgery in February 2016. Since then, I have worked with a trainer, and continue to do stretching, aqua therapy, walking, and bicycling as of this writing.

Now that you've heard my story of my journey through chronic pain and have begun to think about key aspects of your own experience, let's turn next to some facts about chronic pain.

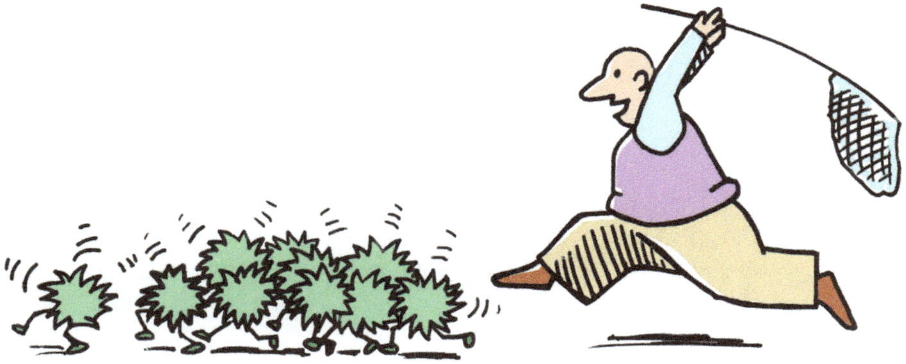

Catching facts proved difficult for slow-footed Melvin.

Chapter 2: Ten Facts About Chronic Pain

Whatever has been your experience, you will realize that you are not alone in having chronic pain. If anything, it is my intention to renew your hope that you can reduce your levels of chronic pain, first, by accepting 10 facts about chronic pain that are common to everyone who has it, and second, by using the strategies I identify in my Pain Management Lifestyle model to become more hopeful that you can reduce it.

10 Facts About Chronic Pain

1. Chronic pain isn't new -- the intensity of the pain is.
2. Chronic pain is subjective.
3. Each person with chronic pain is different.
4. Pain is multi-dimensional.
5. You may always have chronic pain.
6. Some coping strategies are better than others.
7. You must let go of "the way you were" before chronic pain.
8. People with chronic pain differ in their motivation to change.
9. Times are changing rapidly.
10. You are free to determine what is in your best interests to reduce chronic pain.

Choosing A "Pain Management Lifestyle"

Either By

ACKNOWLEDGING IT OR DEFENDING AGAINST IT

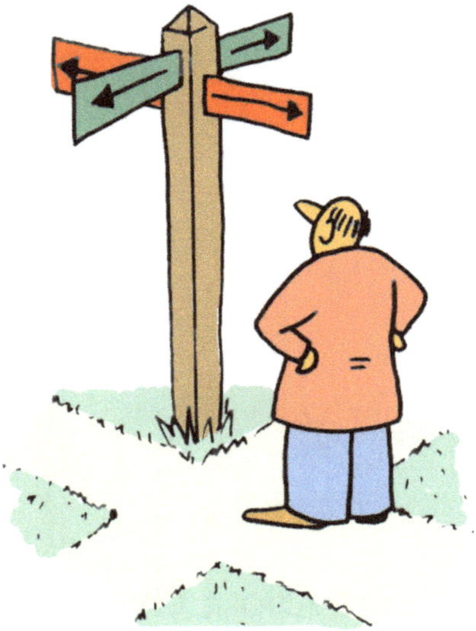

FREE CHOICE!

Fact #1: Chronic Pain Has a Different Intensity

Pain is not new for anyone having it chronically. It's just that the intensity of it is different.

Like other human beings, you've experienced pain since infancy. Often, it's a positive signal that indicates you're hurting; that you need help; that you're hungry, tired or need a new diaper. As you aged, you were pained by something that was hurting. You experienced pain from temporary separations, losses or rejections. Often, your pain was seen as an opportunity to self-soothe, grow, learn to deal with disappointments and frustrations and to delay gratification. You experienced all kinds of emotional pain like anxiety, sadness or anger, and had the ability to reduce your pain by learning language, by saying or doing things that made you relieved. You had pain from life stressors, many of which you had no control over but recovered from.

Then there was pain you developed from faulty thinking or what I'd call "infections" in the prefrontal cortex of your brain. This is where you developed higher-level functioning skills like problem-solving, cognitive shifting or the ability to change your way of thinking when making transitions, and self-reflection. You've had to cope with pain in many ways to build self-esteem, optimism and resilience. Your pain may have increased from not meeting high self-imposed standards or by becoming preoccupied with internal worries over situations you found uncontrollable. Your pain could have come from feeling too much bitterness or guilt, or too little love or affection. You could have pain from abuse.

When you have too much pain, your central nervous system becomes over-sensitized. Even slight touches or pressures can be painful for you if you suffer from fibromyalgia. This is called central sensitization. Your pain can be felt in many places, at different times.

You have the capability to reduce your pain neurologically by utilizing the different strategies I'll recommend later in the book that can alter your neural pathways in positive ways. This is called "neuroplasticity."

Fact #2: Chronic Pain Is Subjective.

Your experience of chronic pain is unique and different from every other person's experience. Everyone has different physical perceptions of pain based on their levels of hypersensitivity and pain thresholds. For example, why is it that one person can't walk fifty feet while another person can hike mountain trails, even though both have the same disc degeneration or bulges in their spinal discs at the same vertebrae levels? Why can someone with stenosis do

Pain Management Lifestyle:

The ability to choose ongoing specific thoughts, emotions and actions that help you to foster resilience when you are challenged by chronic pain.

The ability to reduce your chronic pain using the 5 pain scales over time.

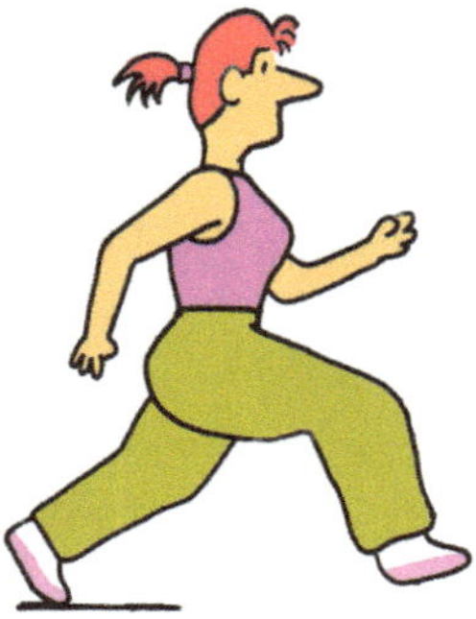

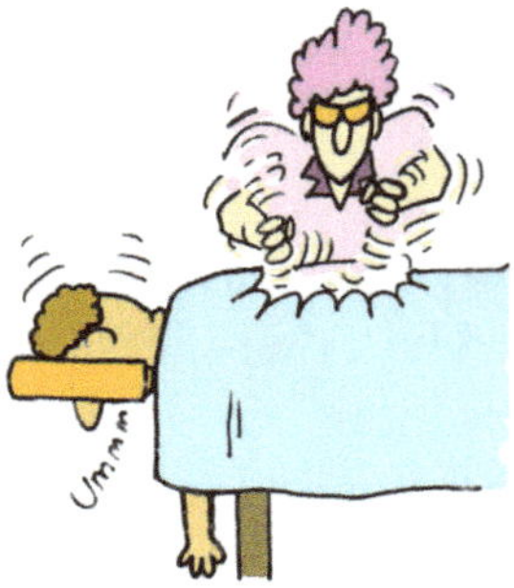

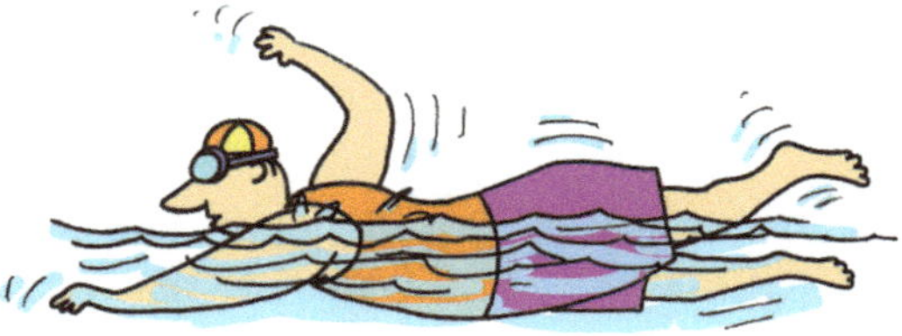

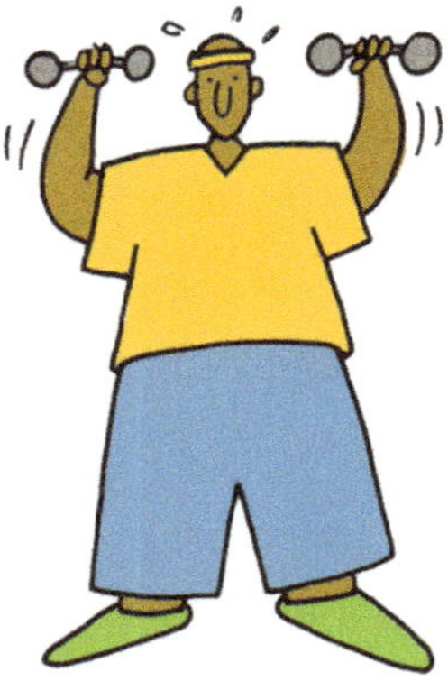

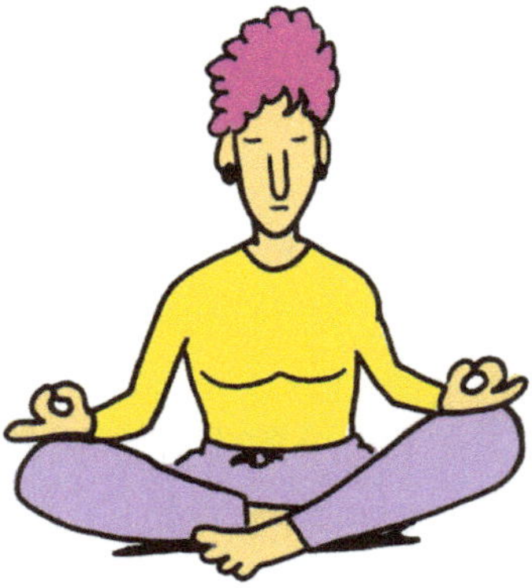

gardening, while another person with the same condition can't even bend down? There are multiple factors that contribute to your experience of pain.

Fact #3: Each Person with Chronic Pain is Different.

Your pain perception is influenced by your genetic predisposition, temperament, and organ system's vulnerability to stress. Your brain segments grow at different rates than other people's. This is especially true for the frontal lobe, which is responsible for higher-level executive functions. This area is similar to the computer processor that regulates how your car functions. Your car's fuel injector is similar to the part of your brain called the limbic system. Each person has different, early developmental experiences in achieving major milestones in speech, and fine and gross motor development. Your exposure to a different parenting style influences your growth, as do your sibling order, family and friend interactions, schooling and cultural background. Your early experiences of trauma, like physical or sexual abuse, can have a markedly high impact on your capacity to cope with pain.

Fact #4: Pain is Multi-Dimensional.

Your pain is generated in many ways. There is your physical pain that the medical community only measures by asking you, "On a scale of 1 to 10, what is your pain level right now?" But what about your cognitive or thinking pain, based on faulty appraisals of situations in your past, or based on negative self-talk? Then there's your emotional pain, such as having different levels of depression, anxiety, anger, and happiness. Your unique appraisal of pain comes from experiencing different life stressors at different times. You have different strengths that allow you to deal with pain, like coping, self-care, self-efficacy or experiencing mastery of completing tasks, assertiveness, optimism, resilience, gratitude, love and spirituality. All these dimensions contribute to your ability to lower your pain. Consequently, you must measure and self-monitor them, even on a weekly basis.

Fact #5: You May Always Have Chronic Pain.

This may be a tough one for you to accept, since any level of pain lasting longer than three months is considered "chronic." You'd like to believe that your physical pain can be eliminated once and for all, but this won't happen because we're describing multiple contributors to your pain that impact you at different times.

If you suffer from chronic pain, instead of ridding yourself of pain once

Some Maladaptive Coping Strategies

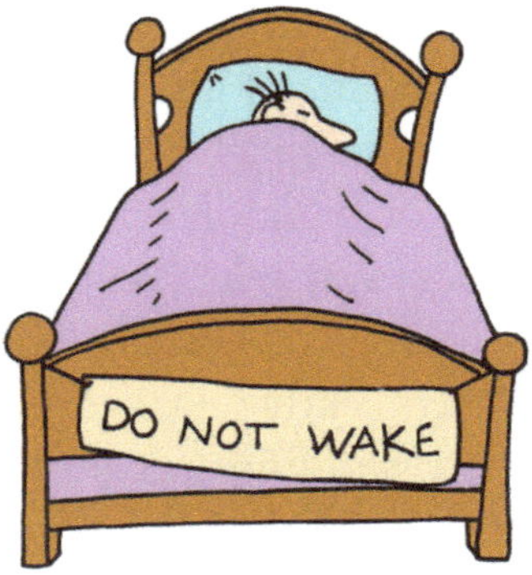

Staying in Bed

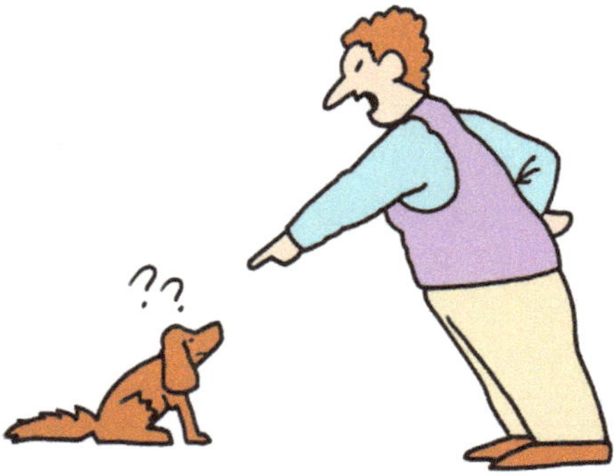

Blaming others

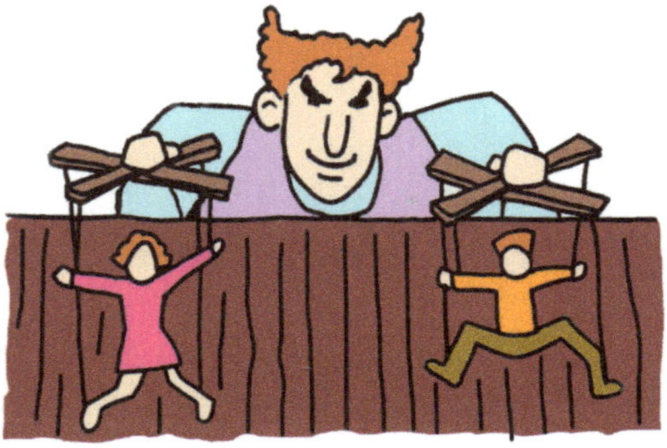

Controlling others

and for all, your goal will be to reduce your negative ratings on the specific pain scales included in this book that measure increased pain, and to improve your positive ratings on scales that show reduced pain, over time. (We'll talk more about these scales in Chapter 4.) This is very similar to the relapse prevention techniques used for people who are trying to maintain realistic weight ranges, or diabetics watching their blood sugar levels, or for people trying to reduce their use of substances like alcohol, tobacco, or opiates.

Fact #6: Some Coping Strategies Are Better Than Others.

There are different ways to cope with having chronic pain. Some are much better than others. If you see yourself using these "coping" strategies, try to stop and find more beneficial ones. *(See Chapters 6 through 11 for ideas.)*

Avoid: You stay away from taking any action that can help you reduce chronic pain. This can simply be staying in bed all day, thinking it's better to just lie there under the covers and escape from experiencing any pain, or you might avoid seeing family or friends.

Rationalize: You come up with all sorts of reasons to not do anything to reduce your chronic pain.

Cover Up: You cover up your feelings by drinking excessively, smoking more cigarettes, eating compulsively or relying excessively on opiates. Anxiety, Depression and Anger: You become more anxious, depressed or angry.

Regress: You regress, acting like a child who is demanding, throwing tantrums, crying constantly, or dependent.

Blame: You blame others for your chronic pain, making them feel less worthy because they've never experienced it.

Play the Victim: You become a victim, seek negative attention, increase your physician visits, or become disabled.

Control Others: You may utilize chronic pain symptoms to have control over your relationships. Symptoms can be very powerful in persuading others to be accommodating to your needs.

Defending

CONSEQUENCE OF MAKING MALADAPTIVE CHOICES
("Stuckness" - Defeatism)

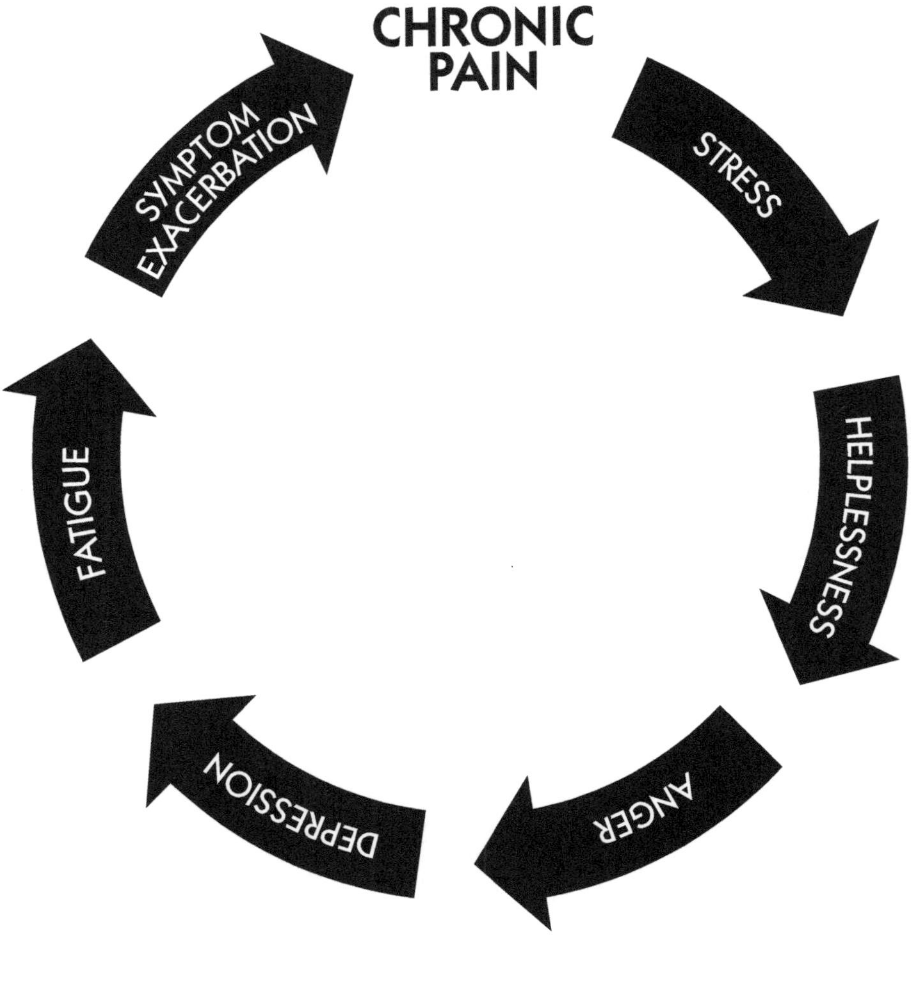

Fact #7: You Must Let Go of "The Way You Were" Before Having Chronic Pain

Grieving, or letting go, of the way you were before having chronic pain is a critical stage to work through.

You can't change why you were given certain life challenges, but you can certainly learn from them. Who said life was fair? It rarely is. But who said mourning isn't healthy? It tests your capacity to build resilience. All hope isn't lost. You may need to lower your standards if you think grieving isn't an acceptable way to cope with loss. You should reappraise your condition by grieving or letting go as a challenge or an opportunity to grow. Even trees lose their leaves in the fall to make way for new ones in the spring. Perennial flowers wither only to blossom more beautiful than before.

The late physician and author Elizabeth Kubler Ross identified five stages of grief that can help you accept your loss rather than remain stuck in denial or continuing sadness. While Dr. Ross identified the five stages as denial, anger, bargaining, depression and acceptance, she did not assume you'd go through each stage with equal intensity or experience each stage just like other people do.

Grief stages may not have a clear progression. Still, each stage has its characteristics. For example, if you experienced a major trauma like a serious injury from a car accident, you might first experience shock, disbelief and a numbing of feelings. You may enter some dreamlike state or escape into fantasy about not having pain. You may even turn to alcohol or drugs to dull the pain. Being angry about having chronic pain is real. You can be angry at the medical professionals who might have misdiagnosed your condition or might have given you poor advice. You can be angry at those who love you for not knowing what it's like to have your pain. You can even get angry at G-d or any other higher power you believe in. No matter who or what you're angry about, the feeling doesn't take away the pain. You may not realize it at the time, but with your anger, you may be pushing away the most important people in your life who love and care about you.

You may want to bargain with G-d or a higher power to get rid of the pain. You may seek greater control of it by going from one health care provider to another, looking for the right answer to allow you to go back to the way you were before the pain began.

You may focus a great deal on what you could have done to have prevented the pain from occurring. You may feel much guilt and regret for being careless in situations that you thought you had no control over. A greater conflict is to be thinking about how life could be if you didn't have chronic pain.

Becoming depressed is normal when you are mourning your old life free of pain. You may feel so alone that you think no one cares. Your closest family and friends may not understand what you're going through because they never had chronic pain. The loss of your previous life is so intense that you may become so depressed that you think it's not worth living anymore. Feelings of helplessness and hopelessness may overwhelm you to the point that you can't move without experiencing pain. You cry, even sob at times, longing to return to those days when you thought nothing about ever having chronic pain.

You can't begin to reduce your chronic pain unless you complete this mourning phase. In her book *Necessary Losses*, author Judith Viorst describes how each of us encounters painful situations throughout life. You need to let go of idealistic and unrealistic expectations that all your pain will eventually be gone. We're talking not only of physical pain but of emotional pain, of pain from faulty thinking, life stressors or lack of fortitude. Sounds like a tough one. Well, it is! No one likes to hear that a more realistic goal is to reduce one's pain than to be totally free of all pain.

Acknowledge

MOURNING – GRIEVING – LETTING GO

"The way one was" vs. "the way one wants to be" vs. "the way one is"

Shock/Denial –
Pain/Guilt
Depression/Reflection
Loneliness

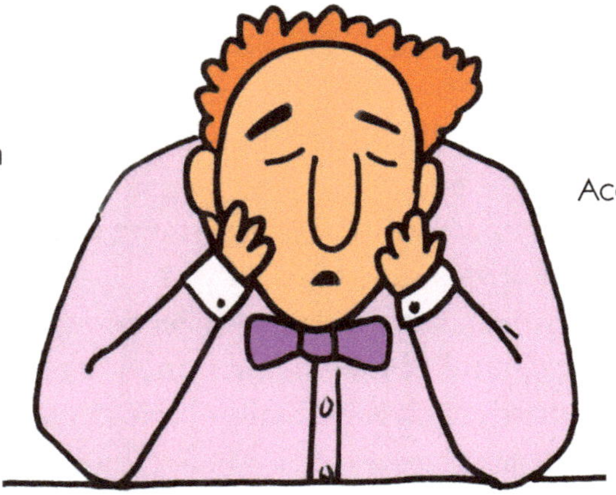

The Upward -
Reconstruction/ Working Through
Acceptance and Hope

Receive — Reflect --- Accept --- Adapt

Fact #8: People with Chronic Pain Differ in Their Motivation to Change.

James Prochaska and Carlo C. DiClemente (1983) designed a "motivation to change" model that is still used today to determine your motivation to change your thoughts, feelings and actions. Their model implies that individuals move through a progressive series of stages, each of which requires different tasks. While it is assumed that you progress from one stage to the next, the authors acknowledge that you can begin at any stage and can move back and forth between stages at any time because of relapses.

The stages of change include the following:

- Pre-contemplation (Denial)
- Contemplation (Ambivalence)
- Determination (Commitment)
- Action (Participation)
- Maintenance (Continuity)

Let's look at each of these stages one by one.

Pre-Contemplation (or Denial) Stage

If you are in the pre-contemplation stage, you deny that there is sufficient reason to change your behavior. You avoid change because you believe your present strategies to deal with pain are good enough, or you're sure someone else thinks you have more of a problem coping with chronic pain than you do. You have no thoughts about changing, even if your coping strategies are unhealthy, like staying in bed; not exercising; or drinking, eating or smoking excessively. You believe you have tried to change your present ways of dealing with pain with little to no benefit. You don't view any alternative strategies as effective based on your past experiences.

In fact, you resist changing your behaviors because the benefits of continuing the strategies you are already using to cope with chronic pain outweigh the negative ones. For example, you may rationalize that it doesn't matter whether you take walks or go regularly to physical therapy. Perhaps you may say something like, "What's the use? My pain's not going away" or "At least I feel relief when I lie down." You can justify maintaining these strategies and you believe that you're doing enough to cope as best as you can. If you're depressed, you experience even more reasons to do less. You're aware others will never understand what chronic pain is like because they've never had it.

If you have increased levels of anxiety, you are clear that remaining at home gives you greater security and comfort than going to the mall for a walk or driving to physical therapy appointments. If you get panic attacks or fear uncontrollable situations, then there are greater benefits to you in avoiding going out. Martin Seligman identified this condition as "learned helplessness." When you believe that whatever you do will only sustain chronic pain, you will give up trying to change to make it better. You will become depressed, and stick to what you are doing.

Sustaining high levels of chronic pain can be worthwhile for some people. There are unrecognized advantages to not changing your present strategies to cope with chronic pain. For example, you can remain depressed because it can be one of the only ways you have to get other people's attention and concern. Having continued pain can be a way to avoid household responsibilities or to control what others say or do around you at home or when out with friends. You can blame your chronic pain on others or come up with multiple reasons why you should not change your pain levels. You can maintain high pain levels to get disability insurance or to file a lawsuit against a person or an institution.

I'll never forget the maladaptive strategies used by a person with whom I played tennis. He obtained Social Security Disability because he was too depressed to cope with an impending divorce. That person wound up selling merchandise "under the table" (meaning the income was hidden from normal reporting and taxation), purchased two ski condominiums, skied every winter and continued to play tennis, all year long. His presumed depression paid off.

Another person came to see me because he was having severe panic attacks. When I asked what he had tried in the past to change his panic attacks, he offered a litany of strategies, all of which "never worked." He never came back after claiming that he wanted to reduce his attacks. Two weeks later, I received a letter from his attorney, asking for a full report of the patient's condition because he had an appeal hearing coming up with the disability board. The patient never wanted to change his condition. His attorney simply told him to see a psychologist to obtain more credible information to help his appeal. I refused and wrote to the attorney that the man was a malingerer.

Don't get me wrong. There are many sincere people who truly have chronic pain that impedes their ability to work and enjoy life. They deserve disability insurance. For example, a middle-aged female school administrator was referred to me for an evaluation and therapy after a hard fall from a rickety school ladder, injuring her left arm and wrist and rendering her incapable of performing administrative tasks. This woman had a clear desire to return to work, missed not being at her school job, and became increasingly depressed. She saw a specialized orthopedic surgeon, then went for physical therapy. Both the surgeon and physical therapist informed the woman that physical recovery would take a long time due to the complexity of her multiple hand and wrist injuries. While she chose to file for disability, she had to grieve the loss because she had a strong work ethic.

Prochaska and DiClemente wrote that one's pre-contemplation resistance to change is identified as the "4 R's": reluctance, rebellion, rationalization and resignation. If you're a reluctant pre-contemplator, you either lack knowledge or simply don't want to change. You may be fearful or reluctant to risk the discomfort of change. If you're a rebellious pre-contemplator, you may know why you don't want to change and don't like being pressured or told what to do. You may like to argue with your medical practitioner or caring other, giving all kinds of reasons to not change. If you're a rationalizing pre-contemplator, you may come up with all kinds of excuses to not change. You minimize harm and have difficulty thinking about the benefits of any change. Finally, if you're a resigned pre-contemplator, you give up and do nothing to change because you believe nothing else will improve your condition (learned helplessness).

The best kind of help for you to get at this stage is consciousness-raising or increasing your awareness by obtaining educational information about your pain condition. You need others to be sensitive and understanding as to why you may not want to change, especially if it means listening to your sadness in grieving what you have lost or the benefits of feeling relief by simply lying in bed. You want others to accept and empathize with what you say while understanding that the decision to change or not change is totally up to you, even if it may be against medical advice. You want them to validate your lack of readiness and to discuss how your current behaviors are influenced by thoughts and feelings about changing, without being judgmental. You want others to affirm that the decision to change is up to you, even if they realize how difficult it is for you to change. You may want to explore specific options like visiting pain websites or blogs to gain more information, or talking to others who've overcome obstacles while accepting that you may still not want to change.

One tool to address the ways you are coping at this stage is to use a scaling method. For example, you may ask yourself, "On a scale of 1 to 10, with 1 being not confident and 10 being very confident, how confident am I that I want to maintain the beliefs I have about changing and the strategies I am using presently to cope with chronic pain?"

Contemplation Stage

In the contemplation stage, you become more serious in your thinking about change. You acknowledge that there is a problem and you weigh the pros and cons of change, but don't yet commit to any action. Instead, you gather more information and are open to further exploration of alternative strategies, weighing their short- and long-term consequences and the pros and cons of change. Often, it is helpful to rate each reason for and against change on a scale of 1 to 5, with 1 not being a very important concern and 5 being a very important concern. You'll end up with two scores. The first is the number of advantages versus disadvantages to change, and the second is in favor of change or to keep doing what you already are doing to cope with chronic pain.

It is helpful for you to gain additional information from important others when doing a sort of cost-benefit analysis of change. Try to accentuate the positive reasons to change your strategies for reducing pain and improving your quality of life. Hear other people's perspectives about your reasons and the weights attached to them for and against change, especially in the long term.

This stage is particularly important to work through if you tend to become anxious often and worry constantly about what to do differently to reduce your pain. Constant worry can lead you to remain paralyzed in this stage. Realize that it is the next stage, the action stage, that will bring you pain relief.

I am still surprised that so many health care practitioners continue to give you advice about what you should do for your pain without considering that you may still be in a pre-contemplative or contemplative stage of change.

Here's an example:

John is overweight and has chronic pain. He doesn't want to go for his yearly physical because the last few times he went, all he could remember was that his healthcare practitioner told him what to do about his weight. But his wife Selma demanded that he go. John scheduled an appointment and reluctantly went to the office.

After the usual check-in routine and ten-minute wait for his practitioner, there was a knock on the door. "Good afternoon, John. It's great to see you again! I know you've been expressing concerns about your constant pain, so I'm here to check you over thoroughly today." John nodded in agreement. The practitioner then checked John thoroughly and said, "You know John, I'm very concerned about your weight and the impact it has on your pain levels. Listen! I want you to get into a structured exercise routine and see my colleague who runs a nutrition program." John agreed.

Eventually, John got dressed and went home. His wife Selma asked him, "So, how did it go?"

"Great!" John said happily. "The practitioner told me that I'm doing fine. My weight is okay and I don't have to come back until next year."

Imagine how much further the practitioner could have gotten if he or she said something like, "Look, John, I understand it's difficult to commit to anything right now. So, why don't we do this? Let me give you some additional information about the relationship between chronic pain and weight. How about after reading this, you make a list on a sheet of paper all the reasons you don't want to do anything about your weight. On the other side, list all the reasons why you may want to do some things about it and indicate the degree of importance each reason has for you, and let's see what you get."

Preparation Stage

In the next stage, the preparation stage, you've reviewed all the costs and benefits of change and now you're 100% committed to action. You design strategies to improve your pain condition. but you don't yet put them into action.

Goal-setting is a major priority at this stage. You make a list of potential goals that would be the most realistic for you to try to achieve. To reduce frustration and disappointment, you should establish goals that are specific and realistically attainable within identified time periods. If your goals are too high, then you should divide them into sub-goals (action steps) to fit the reality of your condition. This is especially true if you are somewhat of a perfectionist who has high self-standards and has difficulty lowering them. You may find it somewhat anxiety-provoking and painful to let go of what you could do in the past, but consider the price you pay for struggling to maintain such high standards, especially if you have been a high achiever and performed exceptionally well in certain areas before you had chronic pain. It is best to establish realistic short- and long-term goals so that you don't become further frustrated and disappointed.

Let's say John decided to do what his practitioner advised and realized that he needed to make that 100% commitment to change. To help himself lose weight, he wrote down the following goals and sub-goals:

1. Eat healthy

A. Have a nutritionist help me get to a better weight range.
B. Establish a healthy amount of weight to lose each month.
C. Buy and eat only healthy foods.
D. Weigh myself each day in the morning.
E. Have Selma and two friends support me in my efforts to lose weight.

2. Exercise

A. Walk each day, starting at 15 minutes. Increase gradually to 1 hour.
B. Join the local gym and go there at least 3 times weekly. Ride stationary bike for 35 minutes.
C. Write down positive self-coping statements to confront all my reasons to avoid exercising.

Once you have your goals written down, evaluate them. How important is it that you achieve these specific goals and what are the reasons? Are these goals written in positive way? Did you define these goals in positive ways? For example, "I will improve my health and feel less pain if I lose X pounds in X months" is much more positive than "I will lose weight so I don't feel like such a fat loser." Are these goals realistic given your pain condition? Could you divide a large goal into smaller action steps to be taken within a specific time frame? Are your standards too high? How will you know that you have reached these goals?

It will be helpful to use the S.M.A.R.T. model when writing down your goals to reduce your chronic pain. Put simply, a S.M.A.R.T. goal is defined as one that is specific, measurable, achievable, results-focused, and time-bound.

- **Specific:** Goals should clearly define what you will do, why you want to do it, and how you will do it.
  Example: *"I will lose 50 pounds, then maintain a healthy weight range over time to help relieve my leg pain. I will do this by eating in a healthy way and by exercising a minimum of 15 to 35 minutes each day."*
- **Measurable:** Goals should be measurable so that you have clear evidence that you have accomplished them.
  Example: *"I will know that I have lost 50 pounds by weighing myself each morning."*
- **Achievable:** Goals should be attainable. They should be realistic and based on your knowledge, skills, and abilities.

Prochaska and DiClemente's Transtheoretical Stages of Change Model

- Pre-contemplation (4 R's)
- Contemplation
- Determination
- Action
- Maintenance

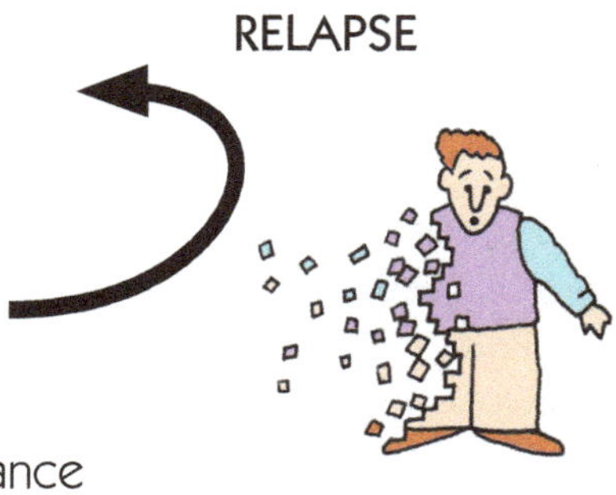

Motivational Techniques To Enhance Change

Express empathy

Develop discrepancy

Avoid argumentation

Roll with resistance

Support self-efficacy

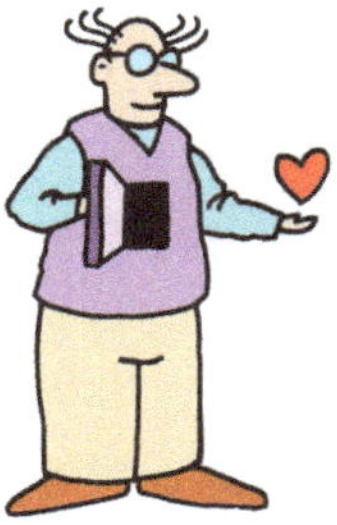

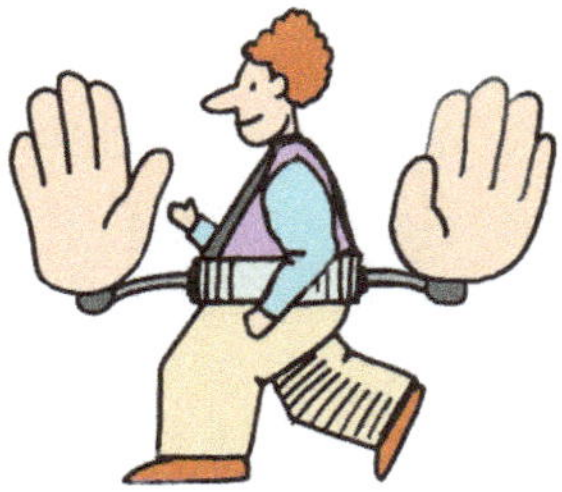

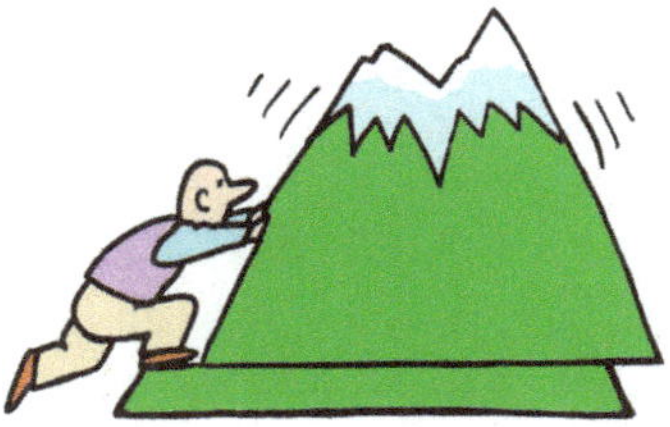

Adapted from materials by Miller, W. and Rollnick, S.

Example: *"I have identified 50 pounds as a realistic amount to lose and, if necessary, I will modify my time frame monthly after discussing my progress with my nutritionist."*

- **Results-focused:** Goals should have measured outcomes.
  Example: *"I will know I have lost enough weight when I lose 50 pounds."*

- **Time-bound:** Goals should be linked to a reasonable timeframe.
  Example: *"I will lose at least 50 pounds in 6 months. I will remain within +/- 5 pounds of my goal at the end of each consecutive month."*

Here are some other goals you may want to consider:

- Identify the triggers that increase your pain.
- Get between 7 to 9 hours of restful sleep per night.
- Identify 10 positive coping statements you can say to reduce your pain.
- List the positive consequences of being at the action stage of change.
- List 10 ways to care for yourself.

When you are considering specific, realistic goals, write down the following:

"I will ________________ by (time frame) __________."

If you are in the preparation stage, you will want to gather information about different strategies that would be in your best interests. Take time to research this as best you can. Educate yourself about what resources are available ranging from books, online information, recommendations from your pain management team and other specialists to help you prepare what you will want to try first.

Action Stage

The next motivation-to-change state, the action stage, is where you can most improve your self-esteem and reduce your pain. Action brings you ultimate pain relief. It is the doing, not the excessive thinking or worrying, that will bring you the most satisfaction and pleasure. In this stage, you experience results.

Each person's strategies to reduce chronic pain are different. You can modify yours at any time, depending on whether you experience continuing success or have too many obstacles. The key is to not lose hope. Stay open to making changes and adjusting your course of action as needed.

It can be very helpful to have a significant other in your life to be a coach or cheerleader or someone else who is also taking action to reduce their chronic pain. The intention is to have someone who offers ongoing encouragement as you pursue your specific chronic pain reduction strategies. That person can provide you with feedback to help you consider whether your goals and sub-goals are still realistic or whether they need to be modified.

Maintenance Stage

Finally, when you are in the maintenance stage, you are continuing to act on your strategies and are aware of any triggers that might cause you to relapse to an earlier stage. This maintenance stage is the most crucial of all because it is ongoing and vital for long-term change. Too many people pursue strategies to reduce chronic pain but don't consider the importance of long-term commitment and the possibility of regressing to previous stages because they experience too little in the way of results. For example, many people who have acted on their goals have reduced chronic pain to a low pain range, but once they get there, their pain levels go back up because they are not fully committed. To prevent relapse, you must pay attention to your thinking and to the emotional and physical triggers that can set you back. Careful self-monitoring of these signals is as important as having an encouraging support network in place.

To maintain a long-term commitment to a Pain Management Lifestyle is to recognize that there will be bumps in the road. Do everything it takes to accept this so that you don't turn around and become frustrated and disappointed, then regress to and remain at an earlier stage. This is why I recommend you continue to use pain scale ratings during the maintenance phase of change, to help reduce your chronic pain long-term.

Fact #9: Times Are Changing Rapidly.

We are witnessing, almost daily, an exponential increase in technological advancements that make it easier to get information and direct activities simply by pushing a button or speaking into a built-in cellphone microphone. While these developments are mostly positive, they have created inherent negative side effects that we can see in individuals ranging from children to adults. Some of these include an inability to delay gratification, tolerate frustration, be patient and/or think critically. We are not being taught or relearning these skills as rapidly as the technology changes. Even adults are ques-

"Pain Management Lifestyle"

Use the the 5 pain scales to monitor the use of any combination of ways.....over time

(Any combination of the items listed below)
"One size does not fit all"

IN COLLABORATION WITH AN INTERDISCIPLINARY STAFF

Surgical Procedures:	Trigger point injections, nerve blocks,epidural steroid and facet injections, neural ablation, implantable pumps, Internal transcutaneous electronic nerve stimulator, surgery
Physical Treatments:	Physical therapy, aquatic therapy chiropractic treatment, orthotics, hot/cold compresses, stretching, exercise, work with a trainer, nutrition for weight loss and maintenance, yoga, tai chi, acupuncture,massage, biofeedback, diaphragmatic breathing, progressive muscle relaxation, herbology, refloxology
Medications:	NSAIDS, acetaminophren, SSRI's, SSNRI's, TCA's, anti-convulsants, opioids, muscle relaxants, topical agents, medical marijuana
Eduation:	Courses, seminars, workshops, webinars, CDs, DVDs, applications, podcasts, blogs, assertiveness training, promoting happiness skills, anger management, stress management, mindfulness meditation, visual imagery, the relaxation response
Therapy:	Motivational interviewing, grief therapy, pain-scale usage and monitoring, cognitive therapy, behavior therapy, distraction, hypnosis, pet therapy, light therapy, aromatherapy, sound therapy, reiki, bibliotherapy-self-help workbooks, journaling, gardening, art therapy, music therapy
Alternative Ways:	Spirituality, prayer, humor, dramatics, socialization

(see detailed list of medications on page 46)

tioning whether they have undiagnosed Attention Deficit Disorder because of sudden, undiscovered problems handling multitask demands. Many individuals are experiencing increased anxiety while others are turning towards addictions if they can't keep up with technological advancements.

Clearly, you are at a critical stage to enhance the executive functions of your brain's prefrontal cortex to keep up with advancing technology. You will need to improve your coping skills, problem-solving abilities and capacities to self-reflect, and think deliberately and critically. Learning to be resilient, optimistic and loving towards others to help reduce your chronic pain supersedes all the tragedy and pessimism you read about every day online or in newspapers.

Fact #10: You Always Have Free Choice To Determine What Is In Your Best Interests To Reduce Chronic Pain.

The ways you eventually choose to reduce your chronic pain will be the best ways for you, even if they aren't what others might prefer. For example, you may find that one of the best ways to maintain your Pain Management Lifestyle is to see a chiropractor twice weekly, have a massage once in a while and walk with a friend twice a week, even if it means walking a few blocks, then stopping to rest, then walking another few blocks. Why is that better or worse than another person who comments regularly on a blog site, does some easy stretches when they get up in the morning, goes to Weight Watchers and joins a beginners' aquatic therapy group? Someone else may find it helpful to practice yoga or tai chi, while another person may benefit from meeting weekly for breakfast with a friend who also has chronic pain. Still another person practices mindfulness meditation daily and has much pleasure in distracting himself from pain by playing the piano or guitar.

It's important for others in your life to not be judgmental or simply give advice on "what is best" for you to help you reduce chronic pain long-term. It is critical for the people around you to be empathetic, to listen and share what they notice about how you're coping with chronic pain.

Choosing A "Pain Management Lifestyle"

Defend **or** **Acknowledge**

FREE CHOICE

Defend	Acknowledge
Avoid	Mourn-grieve-let go how one was vs. how one is.
Rationalize	Accept reality.
Cover Up	Perceive pain as a "challenge" vs. a major loss, threat, catastrophe.
Anxiety	Emphasize resilience.
Depression and Anger Regression	
Blame	
Play the Victim	
Control Others	

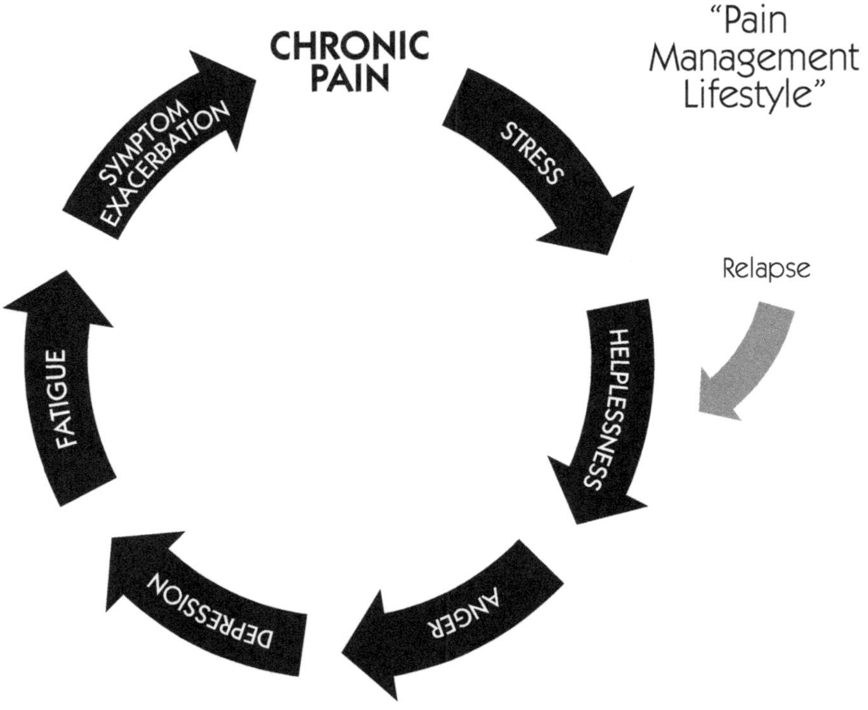

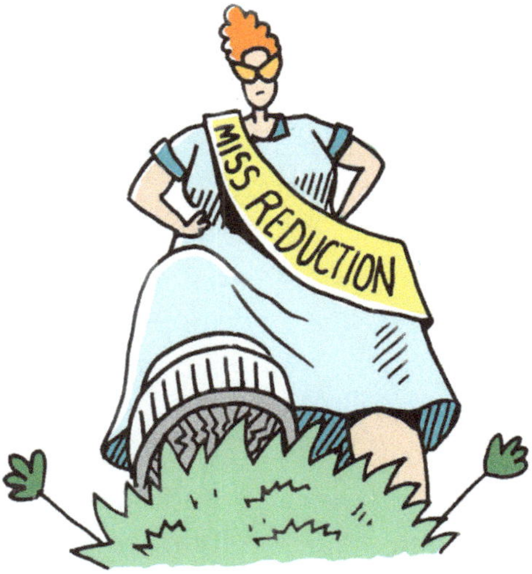

When it comes to pain relief, Miss Reduction puts her foot down.

Chapter 3: A Model to Reduce Pain

My new model for reducing chronic pain grows from the standard question often asked to you by your physician or clinical nurse practitioner, "What is your level of (physical) pain on a scale from 1-10?" Given the subjective, multi-dimensional nature of pain, including multiple factors that contribute to your pain, it is critical to assess and treat pain in a different way. The term "pain" should be perceived as a metaphor for all kinds of pain – not just physical. This is not to diminish the physical aspect of your pain and your desire to try to find a clear, physical reason and treatment for it. Identifying pain triggers and reducing pain requires a holistic approach rather than homing in on one specific aspect like a subjective description of physical pain.

To identify, treat and reduce your chronic pain, you should collaborate with one or more members of your medical team to assess your present condition. This includes your primary care physician, clinical nurse practitioner, and a health psychologist who specializes in pain management. Initially, your primary care physician or clinical nurse practitioner will discuss the reason for your visit and will do all of the following:

- Review your present physical symptoms.
- Perform a thorough physical exam.
- Determine whether your pain is acute (experienced for less than three months) or chronic (experienced for more than three months).
- Request additional medical procedures (like X-rays, an MRI, blood or urine tests) to determine if there is a clear physical diagnosis.
- Refer you to a specialist, like an orthopedic surgeon or neurosurgeon, neurologist or physiatrist, if necessary.

Typically, the cause of acute pain is clear-cut, often resulting from a recent injury. Your pain can be eliminated within a short time period unless a surgical procedure or a recommendation for ongoing physical or chiropractic therapy is required.

If your primary care physician or clinical nurse practitioner decides that your pain is chronic, then you will either meet with the health psychologist who will review your history, then get your perspective about what you think is causing your chronic pain, or you will be referred to a pain clinic where a health psychologist will show how you to complete the five Pain Scales to further assess your present appraisals of your pain in a multi-dimensional way. These Pain Scales measure/assess physical pain, life stress, emotional pain, negative thinking, and fortitude. There are examples of these scales in Chapter 4 with more explanations as to what they measure.

Copies of these scales are available in this book and by sending an e-mail to drgeorgepainless@gmail.com.

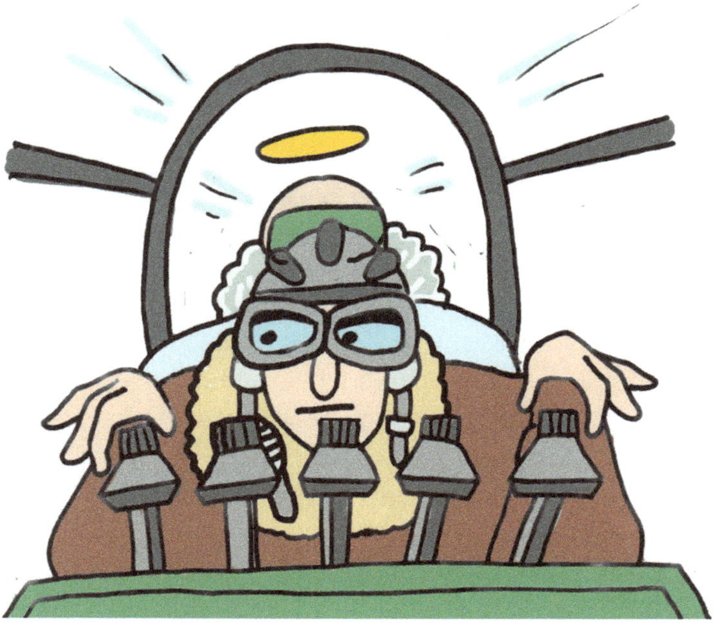

Imagine that you are the navigator in a jet cockpit, monitoring a series of dials that identify the jet engines' efficiency to travel a very long distance *(your life)*. You will want to improve those systems that generate and maintain optimum performance, as indicated by each dial measurement. Each of the five dials measures your physical pain, emotional pain, life stress, cognitive appraisals, and your fortitude *(capacity to handle chronic pain)*.

After scoring and interpreting the five scales with you, the health psychologist will determine what stage of motivational change you are in (as discussed in Chapter 2). If you are in a contemplative stage of change, then the clinician will help you move to the preparation stage by asking you to weigh all the advantages and disadvantages of continuing to use certain maladaptive or ineffective strategies to deal with your chronic pain. Another task will be to help you mourn the loss of how you used to be before the pain existed. The intention is to help you accept that you may always have chronic pain.

Once you enter the preparation stage of change, you are ready to establish realistic, specific, attainable goals, with a major goal being to develop and implement strategies to reduce your negative scale ratings while improving your positive ones over time. If you tend to be a perfectionist and have high self-standards, it will be critical to accept the need to lower your standards a bit by breaking large goals into sub-goals.

Once you are committed 100% to an action plan, then you act to achieve your goals. You will then enter the maintenance phase of change by setting up periodic visits with the health psychologist to evaluate how you're doing in changing your pain scale ratings. You will also discuss specific triggers that can change the pain scale ratings in such a way as to increase, rather than reduce, chronic pain.

There are many ways to reduce your chronic pain. Here are some starter ideas you can might try while collaborating with your medical specialist to see what works best for you.

Medical "Starter Ideas"

- Trigger point injections, nerve blocks, epidural steroid and facet injections, nerve blocks, neural ablation (nerve burning), implantable pumps
- Use of an external transcutaneous electronic nerve stimulator *(TENS device)*
- Insertion of a more sophisticated TENS unit under the skin with electrodes placed at different locations.

Medications

Nonsteroidal Anti-Inflammatory Drugs (NSAIDs)

Aspirin *(Bayer)*, Ibuprofen *(Motrin)*, Naproxen *(Aleve)*

Analgesics

Acetaminophen *(Tylenol)*

Selective Serotonin Reuptake Inhibitors (SSRIs)

Citalopram *(Celexa)*, Escitalopram *(Lexapro)*, Fluoxetine *(Prozac)*, Fluvoxamine *(Luvox)*, Paroxetine *(Paxil)*, Sertraline *(Zoloft)*

Selective Serotonin and Norepinephrine Reuptake Inhibitors (SSNRIs)

Venlafaxine *(Effexor)*, Duloxetine *(Cymbalta)*

Tricyclic Antidepressants (TCAs)

Amitriptyline *(Elavil)*, Imipramine *(Tofranil)*, Clomipramine *(Anafranil)*, Doxepin *(Sinequan)*, Nortriptyline *(Pamelor)*, Desipramine *(Nopramin)*

Anti-Convulsants (Anti-Epileptic Drugs)

Gabapentin *(Neurontin)*, Carbamazepine *(Tegretol)*, Pregabalin *(Lyrica)*

Opioids

Buprenorphine *(Suboxone)*, Methadone, Hydrocodone *(Zohydro ER)*, Oxycontin, Oxycodone *(OxyContin, Roxicodone)*, Hydromorphone *(Dilaudid, Exalgo)*, Morphine *(Avinza, Kadian, MSIR, MS Contin)*, Oxymorphone Hydrochloride *(Opana)*

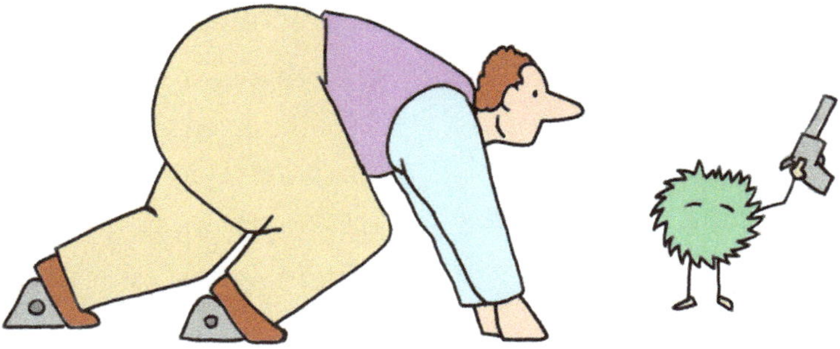

On your mark, ready, set.....

Muscle Relaxants

Baclofen, Chlorzoxazone *(Lorzone, Parafon Forte DSC)*, Carisoprodol *(Soma)*, Cyclobenzaprine *(e.g. Amrix, Cyclobenzaprine Comfort Pac, Fexmid, FlexePax, Flexeril, FusePaq Tabradol, Therabenzaprine-60)* Dantrolene *(Dantrium)*, Diazepam *(Valium)*, Metaxalone *(Skelaxin, Metaxall)*, Methocarbamol *(Robaxin, Robaxin-750)*, Tizanidine *(Comfort Pac with Tizanidine, Zanaflex, Zanaflex capsule)*

Topical Agents

Amitriptyline, Xylocaine, Lignocaine *(Lidocaine)*, Ketamine, DMSO, Capsaicin

Medical Marijuana

Surgery

Physical Therapy

Chiropractic Treatment

Orthotics

Hot or Cold Compresses

Stretching

Exercise

Nutrition for weight loss and maintenance

Aquatic Therapy

Other "Starter Ideas"

Education
(courses, seminars, workshops, webinars, CDs, DVDs, podcasts, blogs)

Assertiveness Training

Promoting Happiness Skills

Anger Management

Diaphragmatic Breathing

Progressive Muscle Relaxation

Work with a Trainer

Yoga

Tai Chi

Massage

Hypnosis

Biofeedback

Acupuncture

Herbology

Stress Management

Meditation
(mindfulness, prayer, the relaxation response, visual imagery)

Cognitive Therapy

Behavior Therapy

Distraction

Socialization
(connectedness, blogs, websites, support groups)

"Bibliotherapy"
(using self-help workbooks)

Art or Music Therapy

Journaling

Gardening

Humor

Dramatics

Pet Therapy

Light Therapy

Aroma Therapy

Sound Therapy

Reiki

Reflexology

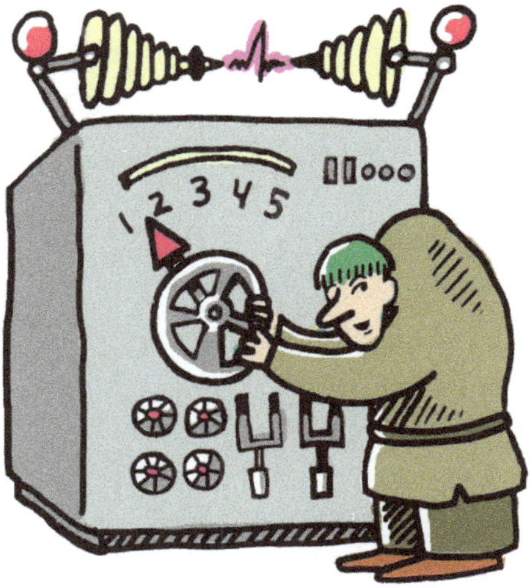

Igor patiently stood by to throw the pain switch.

Chapter 4: The Five Chronic Pain Scales

Once you decide to try some of the starter ideas (like those listed in Chapter 3), it is essential that you monitor how these activities and strategies impact your pain levels. To do this, rate yourself on the five pain scales at least once or twice weekly. Remember that pain is subjective and includes not just your physical pain, but your life stress, your emotional pain, your pain from negative thinking and your lack of fortitude.

You're familiar with the standard medical question "What is your level of physical pain from 1 to 10 (with 1 to 4 being minimal pain and 7 to 10 being severe pain)?" You can rate your level of pain weekly in this same "level of pain from 1 to 10" way for all the scales. Most of the scales (except for the Fortitude Scale) identify higher ratings of 7 to 10 as not being in a healthy range. The opposite is true for the Fortitude Scale and the "Happiness" item on the Emotional Pain Scale, where the higher your rating on these scale items, the better you are at fighting your pain.

Over time, you will want to use strategies to lower your pain levels from 1 to 4 on most of the scale items. You will want to improve your levels from 7 to 10 on the Happiness item on the Emotional Pain Scale and all of the items on the Fortitude Scale.

Using the pain scales will help you remain in the maintenance stage of change and will prevent relapses. If you find that certain strategies are not helpful to you, you can always choose other ones that may be more helpful in reducing your pain levels.

I will provide you with specific ways to improve each of your scale ratings over time in Chapters 6 through 11.

The Physical Pain Scale

The Physical Pain Scale is most similar to the standard, subjective rating scale used presently by the medical community to address how you experience pain. The revised scale featured in this book identifies how daily experiences impact your pain severity by the hour and by period of the day. To use this scale, you will first keep a pain diary by rating your pain experiences on a scale of 1-10 (1 being least painful, 10 being most painful) at each hour for one day, then for three periods of the day for at least two days in one week. The different ratings help identify the activity you are involved in during each rating period, and the location and severity of your pain, using a multitude of different adjectives describing pain sensations. A full week of ratings can help you and your clinician determine certain patterns, like the situations that led you to feel varying levels of pain at certain times of the day. Doing this allows you to generate specific strategies to reduce your pain levels.

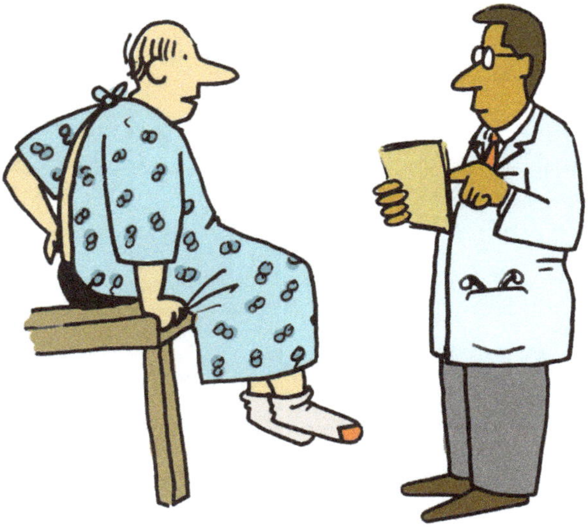

"Not too bad, except that my
heart aches, and a drowsy numbness
pains my senses, feel light-headed,..."

by J.B. Handelsman

Here's an example of a Physical Pain Rating Scale completed by a patient on two consecutive days.

PHYSICAL PAIN SCALE

NAME: Jane **DATE:** 5/24

Please rate your physical pain during the day, per hour, on a scale from 1-10. Please describe what you are doing, the location of the pain, whether it is constant or comes and goes and, what the pain is like using the adjectives on the next page.

TIME: 7:00 am — 1 2 3 4 5 6 (7) 8 9 10 (Low Pain / Moderate Pain / Intense Pain)

Early morning getting up from bed. Pain is in different joints especially right hip aching, agonizing stiff

TIME: 8:00 am — 1 2 3 4 (5) 6 7 8 9 10 (Low Pain / Moderate Pain / Intense Pain)

Having breakfast sitting watching news. Aching all over comes & goes. Aching, stiff, nagging

TIME: 9:00 am — 1 2 3 (4) 5 6 7 8 9 10 (Low Pain / Moderate Pain / Intense Pain)

In Car going to work - joints - upper joints comes and goes Sore - tender - warm

TIME: 10:00 am — 1 2 3 4 5 6 7 8 (9) 10 (Low Pain / Moderate Pain / Intense Pain)

Walking from desk through office Constant multiple joints Pulsing, agonizing, sharp

TIME: 11:00 am — 1 2 3 4 (5) 6 7 8 9 10 (Low Pain / Moderate Pain / Intense Pain)

Sitting at desk - office work. Shoulders, elbows + wrists on both arms. Constant, excruciating, distressing radiating

TIME: *12:00 pm* 1 2 3 4 5 6 7 **(8)** 9 10

Low Pain — Moderate Pain — Intense Pain

Walking to lunch area. Pain comes + goes, radiates to legs. Pins + needles, tingling, stinging

TIME: *1:00 pm* 1 2 3 **(4)** 5 6 7 8 9 10

Low Pain — Moderate Pain — Intense Pain

At desk - taking 5 minute to relax. Pain all over body. Constant Mild, Cool, Tender.

TIME: *2:00 pm* 1 2 3 4 5 6 7 ~~(8)~~ **(9)** 10

Low Pain — Moderate Pain — Intense Pain

After work at desk, Upper multiple joints constant, agonizing, sore distressing

Some words that can help you describe the way your painfeels. Is it ___

Aching?	Cramping?	Taut?	Binding?	Gnawing?
Freezing?	Unbearable?	Heavy?	Hot or burning?	**Nagging?**
Numb?	**Sharp?**	**Shooting?**	Squeezing?	Cold?
Sickening?	Splitting?	**Tight?**	Dreadful?	**Stabbing?**
Punishing or cruel?	**Cool?**	Bolts?	**Tender?**	Throbbing?
Agonizing?	**Excruciating?**	**Tiring?**	**Distressing?**	**Stiffness?**
Pulling?	Flickering?	Pricking?	Pinching?	Stabbing?
Mild?	Intense?	Pulsating?	Intermittent?	Scalding?
Exhausting?	**Sore?**	**Sharp?**	Terrifying?	Killing?
Beating?	Jumping?	Miserable?	Piercing?	Drilling?
Cutting?	Tearing?	Nauseating?	Constant?	Stinging?
Electrical?	Pounding?	Tugging?	Splitting?	Knot-like?
Horrible?	Smarting?	**Pins/Needles?**	**Radiating?**	Waving?
Rasping?	**Annoying?**	Quivering?	Icthy?	Suffocating?
Spreading?	Dull?	**Tingling?**	Grueling?	Drawing?

PHYSICAL PAIN SCALE

Please rate your physical pain for **2 days during the morning,afternoon, and evening** on a scale from 1-10. Please describe what you are doing, the location of the pain, whether it is constant or comes and goes and, what the pain is like using the adjectives on the next page.

DATE: 5/25

Morning **Time:** 8:00am

1 2 3 4 5 6 (7) 8 9 10
Low Pain Moderate Pain Intense Pain

Having breakfast reading newspaper. Aching all over joints - constant - distressing, agonizing & sore

Afternoon **Time:** 2:00 pm

1 2 3 4 5 6 7 8 (9) 10
Low Pain Moderate Pain Intense Pain

at work desk multiple joint pain comes & goes radiating, pins & needles, stinging

Evening **Time:** 7:00pm

1 2 3 4 (5) 6 7 8 9 10
Low Pain Moderate Pain Intense Pain

Laying down in bed watching TV. Multiple joints especially arm & back & neck. aching, pulsating & pinching

DATE: 5/26

Morning **Time:** 7:00am

1 2 3 4 5 6 7 (8) 9 10
Low Pain Moderate Pain Intense Pain

Getting dressed, ate, Multiple joints Constant sore, agonizing, distressing

Afternoon **Time:** 1:00 pm

1 2 3 (4) 5 6 7 8 9 10
Low Pain Moderate Pain Intense Pain

Back from lunch. Pain comes and goes, Mostly neck + arms. tender, sore + aching

Evening **Time:** 9:00 pm

1 2 3 (4) 5 6 7 8 9 10
Low Pain Moderate Pain Intense Pain

Laying down reading. Comes & goes tiring tender + dull.

Some words that can help you describe the way your painfeels. Is it ___

(Aching?)	(Cramping?)	Taut?	Binding?	Gnawing?
Freezing?	Unbearable?	Heavy?	Hot or burning?	(Nagging?)
Numb?	Sharp?	Shooting?	Squeezing?	Cold?
Sickening?	Splitting?	Tight?	Dreadful?	Stabbing?
Punishing or cruel?	Cool?	Bolts?	Tender?	Throbbing?
Agonizing?	Excruciating?	Tiring?	Distressing?	(Stiffness?)
Pulling?	Flickering?	Pricking?	Pinching?	Stabbing?
Mild?	Intense?	Pulsating?	Intermittent?	Scalding?
Exhausting?	Sore?	Sharp?	Terrifying?	Killing?
Beating?	Jumping?	Miserable?	Piercing?	Drilling?
Cutting?	Tearing?	Nauseating?	Constant?	Stinging?
Electrical?	Pounding?	Tugging?	Splitting?	Knot-like?
Horrible?	Smarting?	Pins/Needles?	Radiating?	Waving?
Rasping?	(Annoying?)	Quivering?	Icthy?	Suffocating?
Spreading?	Dull?	Tingling?	Grueling?	Drawing?

The person completing the Physical Pain Rating Scales is Jane, a 46-year-old single female who has a history of having fibromyalgia. She has complained bitterly of chronic pain for many years, having at least 11 tender points that are sensitive throughout her body. She h as chronic fatigue, memory problems, and feels like she has a *"brain fog"* from difficulty with her thinking. She experiences depression and anxiety, has low self-esteem, poor coping skills, and frequent panic attacks. She has settled for a lower-paying job as a day care provider where she has difficulty picking up toddlers and loses her patience easily.

A review of Jane's physical pain scales indicates that she has less pain in the morning, except for overall stiffness upon getting up from bed. Her pain subsides when she is doing self-care activities like having breakfast and being distracted from pain signals by watching the news. The pain remains low while she's driving to work but increases substantially when she walks around the day care facility performing child care responsibilities. Jane's pain lowers substantially when she takes a break to sit at her desk, then increases substantially when she walks around the day care facility, and even when she goes to lunch and then after when she has to stand or she does chores in caring for the toddlers. Taking a five-minute break to meditate at her desk brings some relief but it is not long-lasting, as her pain increases when she performs more demanding job tasks. Her pain subsides only when she can lie down to relax from feeling chronically fatigued.

Jane's pain fluctuates between being constant to coming and going throughout the day. She has multiple pain sites that are indicative of fibromyalgia. It's difficult to read her descriptions of the tormenting pain she feels. Clearly, she is suffering immensely from daily work tasks.

Judging from just her physical rating scales, Jane would do best in a quieter, less physically taxing desk job where she can take frequent breaks while doing simpler, non-physical tasks. The distraction of doing easy tasks would be helpful for her, as would be working in a quieter, supportive environment.

It would be helpful to know if Jane experiences more or less pain based on her doing tasks that require different postures, like bending forwards or backwards. Also, one wonders how long Jane has the strength to walk without pain. A further evaluation by a pain specialist would help determine what kinds of tasks would be easier for Jane to do rather than the ones she is presently doing.

You Try It!

Try keeping a record of your physical pain ratings for a period of at least three days using the sample forms on the next pages, and then use the questions below to help identify patterns of pain or insights about your pain.

- Where is the pain? Do you notice any particular patterns to your pain levels during the day?
- When are the physical pain levels least and when are they most?
- What situations or activities reduce your pain and which ones aggravate it?
- Do you obtain more or less pain from flexing your body than extending it? Are you lifting from your hips or while bending over, thus putting excessive weight on your back?

Based on your responses, can you think of any ways to reduce your physical pain levels just from this rating scale?

PHYSICAL PAIN SCALE

NAME: ____________________ **DATE:** ____________________

Please rate your physical pain during the day, per hour, on a scale from 1-10. Please describe what you are doing, the location of the pain, whether it is constant or comes and goes and, what the pain is like using the adjectives on the next page.

TIME: ________ 1 2 3 4 5 6 7 8 9 10
Low Pain Moderate Pain Intense Pain

____

____

TIME: ________ 1 2 3 4 5 6 7 8 9 10
Low Pain Moderate Pain Intense Pain

____

____

TIME: ________ 1 2 3 4 5 6 7 8 9 10
Low Pain Moderate Pain Intense Pain

____

____

TIME: ________ 1 2 3 4 5 6 7 8 9 10
Low Pain Moderate Pain Intense Pain

____

____

TIME: ________ 1 2 3 4 5 6 7 8 9 10
Low Pain Moderate Pain Intense Pain

____

____

TIME: ________ 1 2 3 4 5 6 7 8 9 10

Low Pain — Moderate Pain — Intense Pain

TIME: ________ 1 2 3 4 5 6 7 8 9 10

Low Pain — Moderate Pain — Intense Pain

TIME: ________ 1 2 3 4 5 6 7 8 9 10

Low Pain — Moderate Pain — Intense Pain

Some words that can help you describe the way your painfeels. Is it ___

Aching?	Cramping?	Taut?	Binding?	Gnawing?
Freezing?	Unbearable?	Heavy?	Hot or burning?	Nagging?
Numb?	Sharp?	Shooting?	Squeezing?	Cold?
Sickening?	Splitting?	Tight?	Dreadful?	Stabbing?
Punishing or cruel?	Cool?	Bolts?	Tender?	Throbbing?
Agonizing?	Excruciating?	Tiring?	Distressing?	Stiffness?
Pulling?	Flickering?	Pricking?	Pinching?	Stabbing?
Mild?	Intense?	Pulsating?	Intermittent?	Scalding?
Exhausting?	Sore?	Sharp?	Terrifying?	Killing?
Beating?	Jumping?	Miserable?	Piercing?	Drilling?
Cutting?	Tearing?	Nauseating?	Constant?	Stinging?
Electrical?	Pounding?	Tugging?	Splitting?	Knot-like?
Horrible?	Smarting?	Pins/Needles?	Radiating?	Waving?
Rasping?	Annoying?	Quivering?	Icthy?	Suffocating?
Spreading?	Dull?	Tingling?	Grueling?	Drawing?

PHYSICAL PAIN SCALE

Please rate your physical pain for **2 days during the morning,afternoon, and evening** on a scale from 1-10. Please describe what you are doing, the location of the pain, whether it is constant or comes and goes and, what the pain is like using the adjectives on the next page.

DATE: ________

Morning **Time:** ________

1 2 3 4 5 6 7 8 9 10
Low Pain Moderate Pain Intense Pain

____

____

Afternoon **Time:** ________

1 2 3 4 5 6 7 8 9 10
Low Pain Moderate Pain Intense Pain

____

____

Evening **Time:** ________

1 2 3 4 5 6 7 8 9 10
Low Pain Moderate Pain Intense Pain

____

____

DATE: ________

Morning **Time:** ________

1 2 3 4 5 6 7 8 9 10
Low Pain Moderate Pain Intense Pain

____

____

Afternoon **Time:** ________

1	2	3	4	5	6	7	8	9	10
Low Pain				Moderate Pain				Intense Pain	

____

____

Evening **Time:** ________

1	2	3	4	5	6	7	8	9	10
Low Pain				Moderate Pain				Intense Pain	

____

____

Some words that can help you describe the way your painfeels. Is it ___

Aching?	Cramping?	Taut?	Binding?	Gnawing?
Freezing?	Unbearable?	Heavy?	Hot or burning?	Nagging?
Numb?	Sharp?	Shooting?	Squeezing?	Cold?
Sickening?	Splitting?	Tight?	Dreadful?	Stabbing?
Punishing or cruel?	Cool?	Bolts?	Tender?	Throbbing?
Agonizing?	Excruciating?	Tiring?	Distressing?	Stiffness?
Pulling?	Flickering?	Pricking?	Pinching?	Stabbing?
Mild?	Intense?	Pulsating?	Intermittent?	Scalding?
Exhausting?	Sore?	Sharp?	Terrifying?	Killing?
Beating?	Jumping?	Miserable?	Piercing?	Drilling?
Cutting?	Tearing?	Nauseating?	Constant?	Stinging?
Electrical?	Pounding?	Tugging?	Splitting?	Knot-like?
Horrible?	Smarting?	Pins/Needles?	Radiating?	Waving?
Rasping?	Annoying?	Quivering?	Icthy?	Suffocating?
Spreading?	Dull?	Tingling?	Grueling?	Drawing?

The Life Stress Pain Scale

Ratings on the Life Stress Pain Scale identify the level of stress you experience for those applicable items that impact your pain levels. You then add them up and divide by the number of items to determine your overall average of life stress, then rate their impact on your family life, work and social functioning. Like the Physical Pain Scale, your ratings are based on subjective experiences ranging in severity from 1 (low) to 10 (high).

Example of a Life Stress Pain Scale

The person completing this Life Stressor Scale is Jim, a 55-year-old married salesman who experienced a major heart attack a few years ago that ultimately led to his needing a quadruple bypass surgery. The high rating he assigned to medical illness as a stressor was not surprising, nor were his ratings of surgeries and aging. He rated job loss high given his history was one of attaining high-salaried, secure positions, then becoming quickly disenchanted with them because he never thought each one was good enough. He gave marital discord a high rating due to his wife being upset that he remained overweight, didn't exercise and was away often each week. Note that his average rating of 4 for major life stressors was inaccurate and well below Jim's actual average of 8.5. Even his low ratings of 3 on the impact of major life stress on his home life, work and family life didn't seem to make sense. This may have resulted from Jim's tendency to minimize and deny, and to usually hold everyone else responsible for his life difficulties. He only sought help for his pain because his wife suggested he do so.

Jim may need help first in becoming educated about how life stressors can impact chronic pain. If he continues to minimize the importance of life stressors because he's in a pre-contemplative stage of change, then it may be best for his clinicians to ask him if significant others are concerned about how he is coping with life stressors and why they are so concerned. It may be further helpful for them to simply empathize and be nonjudgmental with him while reviewing with him the possible short- and long-term consequences of minimizing the impact of his stressors.

LIFE STRESS PAIN SCALE

Please review your present experiences of stress below and rate on a scale of 1-10 the degree to which you believe each stress below impacts your pain.

NAME: JIM **DATE:** 6/28/17

- [ ] Housing
- [ ] Engagement
- [ ] Pregnancy
- [ ] Teenagers
- [ ] In-laws
- [ ] Hobbies
- [ ] Single
- [x] Hours at Work
- [ ] Finances
- [ ] Rape
- [ ] Natural Catastrophe
- [ ] Caring for Elder(s)
- [ ] Legal Issues
- [ ] Insurance Concerns
- [ ] Workman's Compensation
- [ ] Experiencing/ Witnessing/Hearing About Trama
- [ ] Education
- [ ] Relationships
- [ ] Childbirth
- [ ] Parents
- [ ] Friendships
- [ ] Affair(s)
- [ ] Post-Marital Conflict
- [ ] Increased Work Responsibilities
- [ ] Wills/Estates
- [ ] Death of Loved One
- [ ] Lack of Assertiveness
- [ ] Substance Use/ Abuse
- [x] Medical Issues
- [ ] Getting/ Not Getting Disability Insurance
- [ ] Retirement
- [ ] Isolation
- [x] Marital Problems
- [ ] Children's Illness
- [ ] Role Functions
- [ ] Social Life
- [ ] Separation
- [ ] Single Parenting
- [ ] Multi-Tasking Demands
- [x] Aging
- [ ] Grandparenting
- [ ] Religious Affiliation
- [ ] Other Addictions (Porn, Internet, Gambling, etc)
- [ ] Hospitalization(s)
- [ ] Listening to or Watching News
- [ ] Courting
- [ ] Infertility
- [ ] Raising Children
- [ ] Siblings
- [ ] Lack of Exercise
- [ ] Divorce
- [ ] Balancing Parenting and work
- [ ] Career Issues/ Dissatisfaction
- [ ] War
- [ ] Unemployment
- [ ] Verbal or Physical Abuse
- [ ] Getting into an Accident (with/without) injuries
- [x] Surgery(ies)
- [ ] Politics
- [ ] Other: ____________

Please indicate the overall (average) rating of present stress that impacts your pain.

1	2	3	(4)	5	6	7	8	9	10
Not a problem				Somewhat of a problem			A very large problem		

and its -

Impact on Family (1-10)	**Impact on Work** (1-10)	**Impact on Social Life** (1-10)
3	3	3

You Try It!

On the Life Stressor Scale, rate your levels of pain from each major life stressor event. Then calculate your average rating. Finally, what is the impact of your average life stress level on your family life, work (if you are employed), and your social life?

Looking at your answers on the Life Stress Pain Scale, ask yourself these questions:

Do you notice which life stressors impact your pain levels the most?

Do you notice how the average rating of your life stressors impacts the three areas of family life, work, and social life?

Judging from this scale, can you think of ways to reduce any of your life stressors?

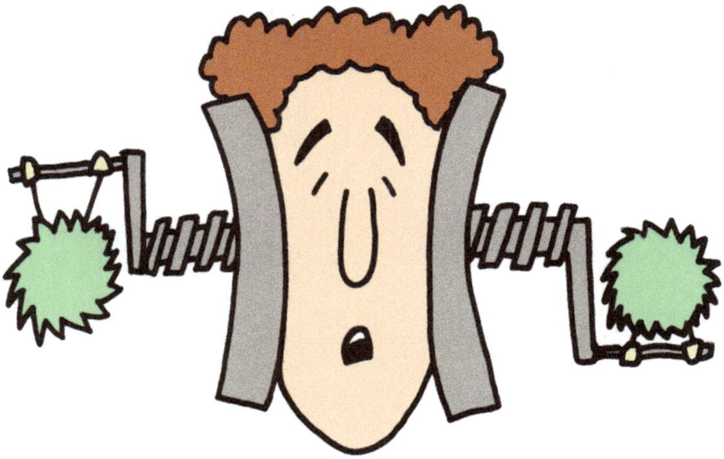

The pressures of life were squeezing the life out of Mort.

LIFE STRESS PAIN SCALE

Please review your present experiences of stress below and rate on a scale of 1-10 the degree to which you believe each stress below impacts your pain.

NAME: ______________________________ **DATE:** __________________________

- ❑ Housing
- ❑ Engagement
- ❑ Pregnancy
- ❑ Teenagers
- ❑ In-laws
- ❑ Hobbies
- ❑ Single
- ❑ Hours at Work
- ❑ Finances
- ❑ Rape
- ❑ Natural Catastrophe
- ❑ Caring for Elder(s)
- ❑ Legal Issues
- ❑ Insurance Concerns
- ❑ Workman's Compensation
- ❑ Experiencing/ Witnessing/Hearing About Trama
- ❑ Education
- ❑ Relationships
- ❑ Childbirth
- ❑ Parents
- ❑ Friendships
- ❑ Affair(s)
- ❑ Post-Marital Conflict
- ❑ Increased Work Responsibilities
- ❑ Wills/Estates
- ❑ Death of Loved One
- ❑ Lack of Assertiveness
- ❑ Substance Use/ Abuse
- ❑ Medical Issues
- ❑ Getting/ Not Getting Disability Insurance
- ❑ Retirement
- ❑ Isolation
- ❑ Marital Problems
- ❑ Children's Illness
- ❑ Role Functions
- ❑ Social Life
- ❑ Separation
- ❑ Single Parenting
- ❑ Multi-Tasking Demands
- ❑ Aging
- ❑ Grandparenting
- ❑ Religious Affiliation
- ❑ Other Addictions (Porn, Internet, Gambling, etc)
- ❑ Hospitalization(s)
- ❑ Listening to or Watching News
- ❑ Courting
- ❑ Infertility
- ❑ Raising Children
- ❑ Siblings
- ❑ Lack of Exercise
- ❑ Divorce
- ❑ Balancing Parenting and work
- ❑ Career Issues/ Dissatisfaction
- ❑ War
- ❑ Unemployment
- ❑ Verbal or Physical Abuse
- ❑ Getting into an Accident (with/without) injuries
- ❑ Surgery(ies)
- ❑ Politics
- ❑ Other:

  ____

  ____

  ____

Please indicate the overall (average) rating of present stress that impacts your pain.

1	2	3	4	5	6	7	8	9	10
Not a problem				Somewhat of a problem				A very large problem	

and its -

Impact on Family (1-10)	**Impact on Work (1-10)**	**Impact on Social Life (1-10)**
___	___	___

The Emotional Pain Scale

Your ratings on the Emotional Pain Scale are simpler than those on the Physical and Life Stressor Pain Scales. On this scale, your clinicians would like to know your subjective perception of how depressed, angry, anxious and unhappy you think you are. Pain may be Inferred from your having high ratings (7 to 10) on depression, anxiety or anger. In contrast, your high rating for happiness would suggest that you feel quite content at this time despite having pain.

It is helpful for you to have a significant other in your life help you rate the four emotional states. That's because another person's perception and perspective can reduce the potential for you to minimize or magnify each emotional state that you are experiencing.

Example of the Emotional Pain Scale

The person completing the Emotional Pain Scale is Vivian, a 63-year-old widow who suffers from severe osteoarthritis in her hips and shoulders. She has been to pain clinics multiple times for trigger point injections and for an ongoing prescription for Tramadol, an opiate that gave her moderate pain relief but that her primary care physician and her clinical nurse practitioner will no longer prescribe because of tightening federal and state regulations. She is not considered a candidate for a full hip replacement surgery given that her X-rays showed only moderate osteoarthritis.

When we look at her responses on the Emotional Pain Scale, it is clear that Vivian's emotional states have a significant impact on her pain ratings. She is severely depressed and lonely, although not actively suicidal, but does admit to having frequent suicidal thoughts and feelings of isolation. Her adult children refuse to be with her because of her frequent complaining and the multitude of angry outbursts she has when interacting with them. Her high anxiety rating is realistic and indicative of her emotional instability and scant motivation to work. Vivian relies only on disability payments for income. She experiences excruciating pain levels and is often at risk for suicide.

Vivian needs much support in dealing with all of her emotional conditions. She may benefit from a prescription for one or several medications to help reduce her chronic stress. Supportive counseling could help her cope and develop further resilience skills. A family intervention might help ease the disconnect between Vivian and her children, and help her develop support networks beyond them.

EMOTIONAL PAIN SCALE

NAME: Vivian **DATE:** 6|28|17

Please review your present experiences of the emotional conditions noted below and rate on a scale of 1-10 the degree to which you believe each one has an impact on your level of pain.

If you have a significant other person in your life please consider asking him/her to help you rate this scale.

(1 = I do not believe this to be true) to (10 = I believe this to be true)

Note: Happiness Scale is scored differnetly than the other three scales-the higher the score, the better the rating.

1. **DEPRESSION:**

1 2 3 4 5 6 7 8 9 10

Low (low-sad-hurt) **Moderate** (unhappy-aggrieved-dejected) **Severe** (depressed-miserable-despondent)

2. **ANXIETY:**

1 2 3 4 5 6 7 8 9 10

Low (concerned-uncomfortable-bothered) **Moderate** (worried-upset-troubled) **Severe** (frightened-overwhelmed-panicky)

3. **ANGER:**

1 2 3 4 5 6 7 8 9 10

Low (annoyed-hurt-disappointed) **Moderate** (frustrated-upset-mad) **Severe** (furious-enraged-incensed)

4. **HAPPINESS:**

1 2 3 4 5 6 7 8 9 10

Low (glad-comfortable-content) **Moderate** (cheerful-pleased-happy) **Severe** (blissful-exhilarated-ecstatic)

You Try It!

Rate your emotional pain levels using the scale below.
Judging from your scale ratings, how do you see yourself coping presently with each emotional state?
What factors do you think are contributing to the impact of each emotional state on your experience of pain?
What is the impact of each emotional state on your relationships with others?
What can you do to reduce your negative emotional ratings and improve your happiness?

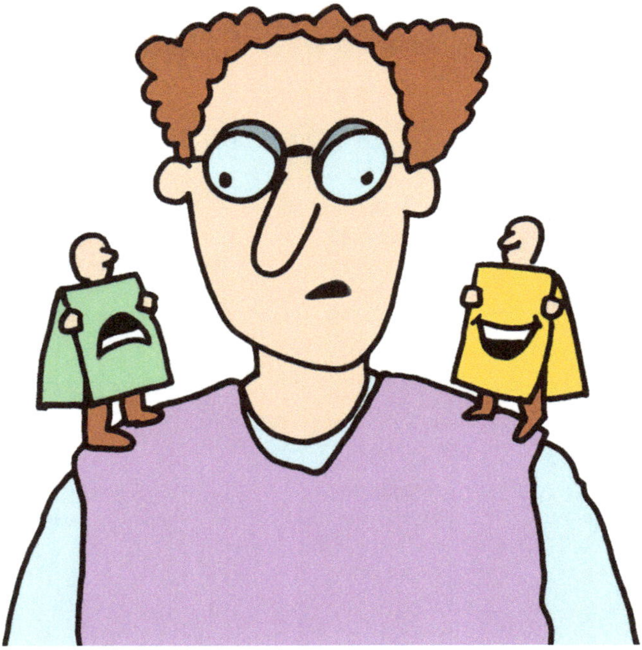

It's a fine line between pain and happiness.

EMOTIONAL PAIN SCALE

NAME: ______________________ **DATE:** ____________________

Please review your present experiences of the emotional conditions noted below and rate on a scale of 1-10 the degree to which you believe each one has an impact on your level of pain.

If you have a significant other person in your life please consider asking him/her to help you rate this scale.

(1 = I do not believe this to be true) to (10 = I believe this to be true)

Note: Happiness Scale is scored differnetly than the other three scales-the higher the score, the better the rating.

1. **DEPRESSION:**

1	2	3	4	5	6	7	8	9	10
	Low			**Moderate**			**Severe**		
	(low-sad-hurt)			(unhappy-aggrieved-dejected)			(depressed-miserable-despondent)		

2. **ANXIETY:**

1	2	3	4	5	6	7	8	9	10
	Low			**Moderate**			**Severe**		
	(concerned-uncomfortable-bothered)			(worried-upset-troubled)			(frightened-overwhelmed-panicky)		

3. **ANGER:**

1	2	3	4	5	6	7	8	9	10
	Low			**Moderate**			**Severe**		
	(annoyed-hurt-disappointed)			(frustrated-upset-mad)			(furious-enraged-incensed)		

4. **HAPPINESS:**

1	2	3	4	5	6	7	8	9	10
	Low			**Moderate**			**Severe**		
	(glad-comfortable-content)			(cheerful-pleased-happy)			(blissful-exhilarated-ecstatic)		

The Cognitive Appraisal of Pain Scale

Your ratings on the Cognitive Appraisal of Pain Scale verify the importance of your understanding the impact of negative thinking based on the works of Aaron Beck on cognitive therapy. Dr. Beck determined the relationship between how you think and how you feel. If you think negatively, you will have increased depression, anxiety or anger. If you think positively, you will feel happier and have less emotional "pain."

As you did on the Emotional Pain Scale, here you should also enlist the help of a significant other to rate each negative thinking error, because your own thinking errors may not be so apparent to you.

Common "thinking errors" around chronic pain include the following:

1. All-or-nothing *(dichotomous)* thinking. You view most situations as falling into one of two distinct categories (always versus never, perfect versus terrible). How often do you catch yourself making statements like these? "I can't work because I always have pain" or "I never feel good."

2. Over-generalization. You reach more global negative conclusions that go well beyond the one situation. Do thoughts like these sound familiar to you? "I can't do what I used to do because I can't bike." "I won't be able to do anything because I can't walk long distances."

3. Mental filtering. You pay more attention to a single detail instead of seeing the whole picture. How often do you think something like, "My pain means that I'm inadequate" or "I couldn't go shopping today means that I'm not good enough"?

4. Disqualifying the positive. You tell yourself that your positive experiences don't count. How often do you think something like, "I was able to cook one meal last night but one night out of twenty doesn't mean much"?

5. Jumping to conclusions (futuristic thinking). You focus on the future and predict it negatively without considering other possibilities. How often do you think something like this? "Oh no! Here comes the pain again. I'll definitely wind up in the emergency room."

6. Catastrophizing (magnification). You exaggerate the importance of negative things and minimize the positive, focusing on the worst-case scenario instead of the best-case scenario. You make a mountain out of a molehill. How often do you think of these kinds of thoughts? "My pain will be totally unbearable" or, "I can't handle this anymore!"

7. Emotional reasoning. You think that if you feel something so strongly, then it must be true. How often do you think negative thoughts like these? "I don't care what my physical therapist says! I feel that it can't be good for me" or "I feel that it's going to be painful."

8. "Should" statements. You hold fixed ideas as to how the world should, ought to, or must be true. (This may relate to your having high self-standards). Do these thoughts feel familiar to you? "I should be able to walk 5 miles." "Everyone should understand why I can't exercise." "I have to take strong pain medications."

9. Labeling. You attach a global, extreme negative label to yourself or to others. Do you often catch yourself make judgments like these? "I'm stupid," or "I'm not good enough," or "All doctors are uncaring jerks."

10. Need for control. You believe that you must control everything in your life: yourself, your relationships, your emotions, or your personal situations. Do you often find yourself having thoughts like these? "I need to know everything about what's going to happen." "The need to control helps me to not feel helpless and powerless."

11. Over-personalization. You believe you're responsible for negative situations and that it is all your fault, even when there is no evidence to indicate that this is true. How often do you catch yourself thinking statements like these? "This pain is punishment for something I did wrong." "If I didn't have pain, then my spouse wouldn't be mad at me."

12. Underestimating your strengths. You minimize the positive traits you have that can help you handle your pain. How often do you have these kinds of thoughts? "I can't handle my pain," or "It's not worth trying anymore."

How to Use the Cognitive Appraisal of Pain Scale to Determine How Much Your Thinking Can Make You Feel Anxious or Depressed

The Cognitive Appraisal of Pain Scale can identify common patterns for people who suffer from heightened anxiety or depression. If you're someone who has a high anxiety level, you may score higher in certain cognitive appraisals than others. Of particular interest is your rating on the control scale, since anxious people value security and have a difficult time feeling uncertain or helpless about situations. Your "need for control" rating may be high if you are a perfectionist with high self-standards. The same is true for "should" statements because, if you are highly anxious, you may invest a lot of energy in what you "should" be doing, but can't do, because of you have chronic pain.

If you rate high on both Futuristic Thinking and Catastrophic Thinking, you're probably a person who worries constantly about a pessimistic future rather than being relaxed enough to enjoy each moment in time or thinking about the probability of positive future outcomes. While future planning is a healthy skill, an overemphasis on the future can elicit feelings of doubt and uncertainty that can parallel a higher-scaled score in the need for control scale.

You may often perceive situations in all-or-nothing, black-and-white ways rather than taking into account the large grey area between extremes. Again, this is true if you are a perfectionist. Perhaps some of these statements sound familiar to you? "I'm either pain-free or in severe pain." "I have to be perfect or I'm inadequate." "I have to do exceedingly well." "I'm terrible."

If you're very depressed, you may often disqualify the positive appraisals of a situation. It is easier for you to think your experiences will "always" be negative and "never" positive. You may make overgeneralizations from one situation to every situation and may tend to filter in only negative conditions about it. You may make mountains out of molehills. Your future can seem catastrophic to you, without any appreciation for the possible positive outcomes, and you have trouble reframing your future as an opportunity or challenge instead of a disaster. If you are depressed, you can be very hard on yourself.

Perfectionists often become depressed if they can't meet high self-standards. If you personalize or see yourself at fault excessively, you may often blame yourself and feel over-responsible, even in situations for which responsibility should be attributed to others or over which you have no control.

Example of the Cognitive Appraisal of Pain Scale

The person completing this scale is Wilson, a 45-year-old divorced man with a long history of chronic pain. He became severely depressed after being involved in a highly conflictual divorce that led to his estrangement from his three daughters, who perceived him as mentally unstable. His former wife disregarded how much pain Wilson had experienced from working so much, leaving little time for his family life. Wilson didn't exercise much, which led to his being overweight and having more pain.

Most of his ratings for negative cognitive appraisals are high, indicating extreme preoccupation with internal thoughts that render him extremely anxious and depressed. He is paralyzed by having so many thinking errors because of sitting around most of the day, doing very little to distract himself, except for work and watching TV.

When asked what he does to help his chronic pain, Wilson often gives all kinds of reasons for not doing anything. It is easy to see why he is so depressed and anxious. He relies excessively on obsessing, rather than considering the impact of his having so many high negative cognitive appraisals on his pain scale.

How might Wilson get help and improve his situation? Given the extent of Wilson's high ratings on this scale, the best treatment would be to help him identify many activities that could distract him from being so focused on having so many negative thoughts. He could reduce both his anxiety and his depression by taking an interest in helping others, doing volunteer work or learning to play a musical instrument – in short, doing anything that takes him outside of himself and his tendency to overthink.

COGNITIVE APPRAISAL OF PAIN SCALE

NAME: WILSON DATE: 6/5/17

Please these different cognitive appraials and rate on a scale of 1-10 the degree to which you believe each appraisal to be true for you.

If you have a significant other person in your life please consider asking him/her to help you rate this scale.

(1 = I do not believe this to be true) to (10 = I believe this to be true)

1. **ALL OR NOTHING THINKING (Dichotomous Thinking):**
   You view most situations as two distinct categories (always vs. never, perfect vs. terrible)
   "I can't work because I always have pain." " I never feel good."
   1 2 3 4 5 6 7 8 9 10
   A little Some A Lot
2. **OVER GENERALIZATION:**
   You make global negative conclusions that go well beyond the one situation.
   "I can't do what I used to do because I can't bike." "I won't be able to do anything because I can't walk long distances."
   1 2 3 4 5 6 7 8 9 10
   A little Some A Lot
3. **MENTAL FILTERING:**
   You pay more attention to a single detail instead of seeing the whole picture.
   "My pain means that I'm inadequate."
   1 2 3 4 5 6 7 8 9 10
   A little Some A Lot
4. **DISQUALIFYING THE POSITIVE:**
   You tell yourself that positive experiences don't count.
   "I was able to cook one meal last night but one night out of twenty doesn't mean much."
   1 2 3 4 5 6 7 8 9 10
   A little Some A Lot
5. **JUMPING TO CONCLUSIONS - FUTURISTIC THINKING:**
   You focus on the the future and predict it negatively without considering other possibilities.
   "Oh no! Here comes the pain again. I'll definitely wind up in the emergency room."
   1 2 3 4 5 6 7 8 9 10
   A little Some A Lot
6. **CATASTROPHIZING - MAGNIFICATION:**
   You exaggerate the importance of things and minimize the positive, you think of the worst versus the best case scenario. You make a mountain out of a molehill.
   "My pain will be totally unbearable."
   1 2 3 4 5 6 7 8 9 10
   A little Some A Lot

7. **EMOTIONAL REASONING:**
You think that if you feel something so strongly, then it must be true.
"I don't care what my physical therapist says! I feel it can't be good for me."
"I feel that it's going to be painful."

1	2	3	4	5	6	7	8	9	10
A little				Some					A Lot

8. **"SHOULD" STATEMENTS:**
You hold fixed ideas as to how the world should, ought to, or must be true. (May relate to high self-standards.)
"I should be able to walk 5 miles." "Everyone should understand why I can't exercise."
"I only need pain medications."

1	2	3	4	5	6	7	8	9	10
A little				Some					A Lot

9. **LABELING:**
You attach a global extreme negative label to yourself or others.
"I'm stupid." " I not good enough." "All doctors ae uncaring jerks."

1	2	3	4	5	6	7	8	9	10
A little				Some					A Lot

10. **NEED FOR CONTROL:**
You believe that you must control everything in your life; yourself, relationships, emotions, or situations.
"I need to know everything about what's going to happen."
"The need to control helps me to not feel helpless and powerless."

1	2	3	4	5	6	7	8	9	10
A little				Some					A Lot

11. **PERSONALIZATION:**
You believe you're responsible for negative situations and that it is all your fault, even when there is no evidence to indicate this.
"The pain is punishment for something I did wrong."
"If I don't have pain then my spouse wouldn't be mad at me."

1	2	3	4	5	6	7	8	9	10
A little				Some					A Lot

12. **UNDERESTIMATING YOUR STRENGTHS:**
You minimize the positive traits that you have to handle your pain.
"I can't handle it." "It's not worth trying anymore."

1	2	3	4	5	6	7	8	9	10
A little				Some					A Lot

Adapted by the author from materials by Aaron Beck, MD

You Try It!

As you fill out the Cognitive Appraisal of Pain Scale, rate the impact of each way of negative thinking on your pain levels. Enlist the help of a significant other to do this, if possible.

Do you notice how any of the negative cognitive appraisals impact your pain?

Do you notice any particular patterns?

Can you come up with any rational responses to your high-rated negative ways of thinking when you catch yourself thinking or saying any of them?

Do you notice any relationship between your pain level ratings on your Emotional Pain Scale and this one?

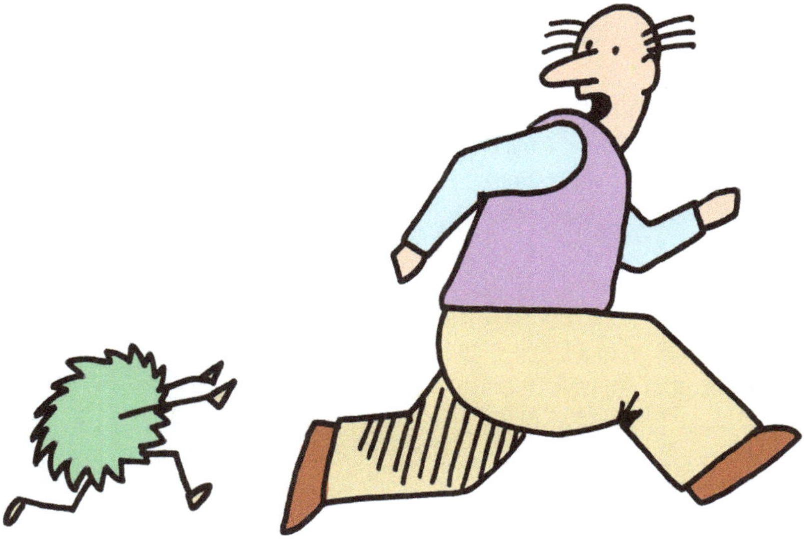

No matter how fast Sy ran, pain was catching up to him.

COGNITIVE APPRAISAL OF PAIN SCALE

NAME: ______________________ **DATE:** ____________________

Please these different cognitive appraials and rate on a scale of 1-10 the degree to which you believe each appraisal to be true for you.

If you have a significant other person in your life please consider asking him/her to help you rate this scale.

(1 = I do not believe this to be true) to (10 = I believe this to be true)

1. **ALL OR NOTHING THINKING (Dichotomous Thinking):**
You view most situations as two distinct categories (always vs. never, perfect vs. terrible)
"I can't work because I always have pain." " I never feel good."
1 2 3 4 5 6 7 8 9 10
A little Some A Lot

2. **OVER GENERALIZATION:**
You make global negative conclusions that go well beyond the one situation.
"I can't do what I used to do because I can't bike." "I won't be able to do anything because I can't walk long distances."
1 2 3 4 5 6 7 8 9 10
A little Some A Lot

3. **MENTAL FILTERING:**
You pay more attention to a single detail instead of seeing the whole picture.
"My pain means that I'm inadequate."
1 2 3 4 5 6 7 8 9 10
A little Some A Lot

4. **DISQUALIFYING THE POSITIVE:**
You tell yourself that positive experiences don't count.
"I was able to cook one meal last night but one night out of twenty doesn't mean much."
1 2 3 4 5 6 7 8 9 10
A little Some A Lot

5. **JUMPING TO CONCLUSIONS - FUTURISTIC THINKING:**
You focus on the the future and predict it negatively without considering other possibilities.
"Oh no! Here comes the pain again. I'll definitely wind up in the emergency room."
1 2 3 4 5 6 7 8 9 10
A little Some A Lot

6. **CATASTROPHIZING - MAGNIFICATION:**
You exaggerate the importance of things and minimize the positive, you think of the worst versus the best case scenario. You make a mountain out of a molehill.
"My pain will be totally unbearable."
1 2 3 4 5 6 7 8 9 10
A little Some A Lot

7. **EMOTIONAL REASONING:**
   You think that if you feel something so strongly, then it must be true.
   "I don't care what my physical therapist says! I feel it can't be good for me."
   "I feel that it's going to be painful."

1	2	3	4	5	6	7	8	9	10
A little				Some					A Lot

8. **"SHOULD" STATEMENTS:**
   You hold fixed ideas as to how the world should, ought to, or must be true. (May relate to high self-standards.)
   "I should be able to walk 5 miles." "Everyone should understand why I can't exercise."
   "I only need pain medications."

1	2	3	4	5	6	7	8	9	10
A little				Some					A Lot

9. **LABELING:**
   You attach a global extreme negative label to yourself or others.
   "I'm stupid." " I not good enough." "All doctors ae uncaring jerks."

1	2	3	4	5	6	7	8	9	10
A little				Some					A Lot

10. **NEED FOR CONTROL:**
    You believe that you must control everything in your life; yourself, relationships, emotions, or situations.
    "I need to know everything about what's going to happen."
    "The need to control helps me to not feel helpless and powerless."

1	2	3	4	5	6	7	8	9	10
A little				Some					A Lot

11. **PERSONALIZATION:**
    You believe you're responsible for negative situations and that it is all your fault, even when there is no evidence to indicate this.
    "The pain is punishment for something I did wrong."
    "If I don't have pain then my spouse wouldn't be mad at me."

1	2	3	4	5	6	7	8	9	10
A little				Some					A Lot

12. **UNDERESTIMATING YOUR STRENGTHS:**
    You minimize the positive traits that you have to handle your pain.
    "I can't handle it." "It's not worth trying anymore."

1	2	3	4	5	6	7	8	9	10
A little				Some					A Lot

Adapted by the author from materials by Aaron Beck, MD

The Fortitude Scale

Over the past few decades, there has been a major shift in the field of psychology towards emphasizing one's strengths. Professionals like Martin Seligman have conducted much research to indicate the positive impact of lessening "pain" by building positivity, optimism, happiness, and resilience (the ability to bounce back from hardships or setbacks). Research has demonstrated that the critical factor that keeps people alive who are taken prisoner during wartime or held hostage by terrorists is their sustaining hope. Building hope rests with a commitment to action and the ability to reframe pain as a challenge rather than a curse.

To take advantage of this research, I designed the Fortitude Scale to help you subjectively rate your strengths that can help you to reduce chronic pain. To do this, you must regain old or learn new coping skills and build your self-esteem by improving your level of self-care and self-efficacy. Increasing your resilience is just as important as learning to be more assertive and think flexibly, to self-monitor well, and to problem-solve effectively. Who wouldn't find humor comforting, mindfulness meditation rewarding, and sustaining optimism helpful? Being grateful for what you have, however simple, is a necessity to contemplate on a daily basis, as is your ability to love others no matter how severe your experience of pain. Finally, there is "Emuna" or your unconditional faith in G-d or a higher power.

The items listed on the Fortitude Scale are as follows:

1. Coping skills: "You can handle it."
2. Self-esteem: "Feeling good about yourself."
    A Self-care skills: "Take care of yourself,"
    B. Self-efficacy skills: "Accomplish things."
3. Assertiveness skills: "Stand up for your rights."
4. Exercise skills: "Just do it."
5. Distraction skills: "Take the time to smell the roses."
6. Mindfulness skills: "Be here now."
7. Problem-solving skills:
    "What is your problem?"
    "What are some of your plans?"
    "What is the best plan?"
    "Act on your plan."
    "How did you do?"
8. Self-monitoring skills: "Think before you act."

9. Cognitive flexibility skills: "Go with the flow."
10. Optimism skills: "Hope for the future."
11. Humor skills: "Laugh and the world laughs with you."
12. Resiliency skills: "You can bounce back."
13. Gratitude skills: "Be thankful for what you have."
14. Supportive system skills: "Connect with family, friends and community."
15. Loving skills: "Do unto others as you would have them do unto you."
16. Spirituality skills: "Emuna" -- one's unconditional faith in G-d" *(or a higher power)*.

Example of a Fortitude Scale

The person completing the Fortitude Scale is Susan, a 32-year-old married woman who works full-time in the medical profession. She often works overtime in high-stress situations, leading her to experience severe back pain and periodic tension headaches. She shows fantastic strengths in many areas based on her Fortitude Scale ratings. For example, she has a balanced level of self-esteem between self-care and self-efficacy, an excellent ability to assert herself when necessary, and a healthy ability to distract herself with hobbies like gardening, yoga, and playing the piano. Susan practices mindfulness meditation each morning and enjoys watching comedies rather than the news that is full of negativity. Of critical importance is her level of gratitude, her love for others (including her devoted network of family and friends), and her passionate love for G-d, based on her religious upbringing.

Where she falls short is in her ability to problem-solve and shift into doing new tasks when she is focusing on current ones. In addition, she needs help with building resilience (the ability to bounce back from hardships). Susan needs help in improving her brain's executive functions, particularly the sequence of problem-solving effectively including problem recognition, cause-and-effect reasoning, and self-monitoring skills. Helping her identify her values, interests, and abilities would prove useful, as would reflecting on how she was able to bounce back from former upsets. Of particular concern will be helping her recognize the positive impact of her overall high Fortitude Scale ratings and using these skills to reduce her chronic pain.

FORTITUDE SCALE

NAME: SUSAN **DATE:** 6|26|17

Please review your present experiences of the conditions noted below and rate on a scale of 1-10 the degree to which you believe each condition has an impact on your level of pain.

Note: The higher the rating, the stronger the belief.

If you have a significant other person in your life please consider asking him/her to help you rate this scale.
(1 = I do not believe this to be true to (10 = I believe this to be true)

1. **COPING SKILLS:** "You can handle it"
   1 2 3 (4) 5 6 7 8 9 10
   Low **Moderate** **High**

2. **SELF-ESTEEM:** "Feel good about yourself"
   Balance between

   A. SELF-CARE SKILLS "You can handle it"
   1 2 3 4 (5) 6 7 8 9 10
   Low **Moderate** **High**

   And B.. SELF-EFFICACY SKILLS "Accomplish things"
   1 2 3 4 (5) 6 7 8 9 10
   Low **Moderate** **High**

3. **ASSSERIVENESS SKILLS:** "Stand up for your rights"
   1 2 3 4 5 6 7 8 (9) 10
   Low **Moderate** **High**

4. **EXERCISE SKILLS:** "Just do it!"
   1 2 3 (4) 5 6 7 8 9 10
   Low **Moderate** **High**

5. **DISTRACTION SKILLS:** "Take the time to smell the roses"
   1 2 3 4 5 6 (7) 8 9 10
   Low **Moderate** **High**

6. **MINFULNESS SKILLS:** "Be here now!"
   1 2 3 4 5 6 (7) 8 9 10
   Low **Moderate** **High**

7. **PROBLEM SOLVING SKILLS:** "What is your problem?""What are some of your plans?" "What is the best plan?"" Act on your plan""How did you do?"
   1 2 3 (4) 5 6 7 8 9 10
   Low **Moderate** **High**

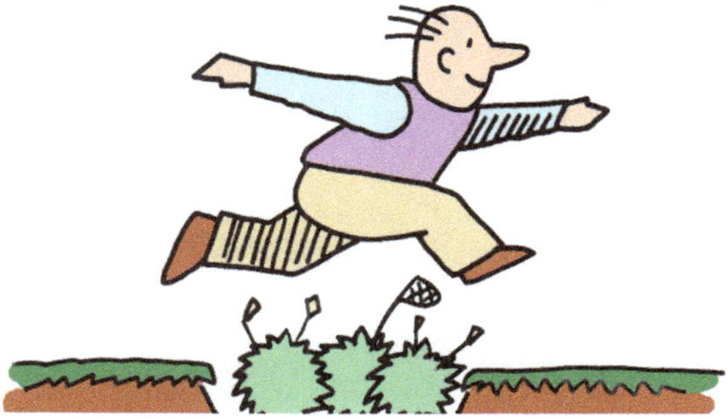

You can leap over the forces of pain.

8. **SELF-MONITORING SKILLS:** "Think before you act"
   1 2 3 4 5 6 7 8 9 10
   Low — Moderate — High

9. **COGNITIVE FLEXIBILITY SKILLS:** "Go with the flow"
   1 2 3 4 5 6 7 8 9 10
   Low — Moderate — High

10. **OPTIMISM SKILLS:** "Hope for the future"
    1 2 3 4 5 6 7 8 9 10
    Low — Moderate — High

11. **HUMOR SKILLS:** "Laugh and the whole world laughs with you"
    1 2 3 4 5 6 7 8 9 10
    Low — Moderate — High

12. **RESILIENCY SKILLS:** "You can bounce back"
    1 2 3 4 5 6 7 8 9 10
    Low — Moderate — High

13. **GRATITUDE SKILLS:** "Be thankful for what you have"
    1 2 3 4 5 6 7 8 9 10
    Low — Moderate — High

14. **SUPPORTIVE SYSTEM SKILLS:** "Connect with family, friends and community"
    1 2 3 4 5 6 7 8 9 10
    Low — Moderate — High

15. **LOVING SKILLS:** "Do unto others as you would have them do unto you"
    1 2 3 4 5 6 7 8 9 10
    Low — Moderate — High

16. **SPIRITUALITY SKILLS:** Emuna "One's unconditional faith in G-d" (or higher power)
    1 2 3 4 5 6 7 8 9 10
    Low — Moderate — High

FORTITUDE SCALE

NAME: ______________________ **DATE:** ____________________

Please review your present experiences of the conditions noted below and rate on a scale of 1-10 the degree to which you believe each condition has an impact on your level of pain.

Note: The higher the rating, the stronger the belief.

If you have a significant other person in your life please consider asking him/her to help you rate this scale.
(1 = I do not believe this to be true to (10 = I believe this to be true)

1. **COPING SKILLS:** "You can handle it"
   1 2 3 4 5 6 7 8 9 10
   Low **Moderate** **High**
2. **SELF-ESTEEM:** "Feel good about yourself"
   Balance between

   A. SELF-CARE SKILLS "You can handle it"
   1 2 3 4 5 6 7 8 9 10
   Low **Moderate** **High**

   And B.. SELF-EFFICACY SKILLS "Accomplish things"
   1 2 3 4 5 6 7 8 9 10
   Low **Moderate** **High**
3. **ASSSERIVENESS SKILLS:** "Stand up for your rights"
   1 2 3 4 5 6 7 8 9 10
   Low **Moderate** **High**
4. **EXERCISE SKILLS:** "Just do it!"
   1 2 3 4 5 6 7 8 9 10
   Low **Moderate** **High**
5. **DISTRACTION SKILLS:** "Take the time to smell the roses"
   1 2 3 4 5 6 7 8 9 10
   Low **Moderate** **High**
6. **MINFULNESS SKILLS:** "Be here now!"
   1 2 3 4 5 6 7 8 9 10
   Low **Moderate** **High**
7. **PROBLEM SOLVING SKILLS:** "What is your problem?""What are some of your plans?" "What is the best plan?"" Act on your plan""How did you do?"
   1 2 3 4 5 6 7 8 9 10
   Low **Moderate** **High**

You Try It!

Please take some time to rate your fortitude scales with the help of a significant other in your life. Someone close to you may be able to recognize your strengths more easily than you can, especially if you have a tendency to minimize them.

What are your strengths and how do they help you reduce chronic pain?

What are the areas that you need to strengthen to help you reduce your pain?

Can you think of ways to strengthen these areas?

8. SELF-MONITORING SKILLS: "Think before you act"

1	2	3	4	5	6	7	8	9	10
Low				**Moderate**					**High**

9. COGNITIVE FLEXIBILITY SKILLS: "Go with the flow"

1	2	3	4	5	6	7	8	9	10
Low				**Moderate**					**High**

10. OPTIMISM SKILLS: "Hope for the future"

1	2	3	4	5	6	7	8	9	10
Low				**Moderate**					**High**

11. HUMOR SKILLS: "Laugh and the whole world laughs with you"

1	2	3	4	5	6	7	8	9	10
Low				**Moderate**					**High**

12. RESILIENCY SKILLS: "You can bounce back"

1	2	3	4	5	6	7	8	9	10
Low				**Moderate**					**High**

13. GRATITUDE SKILLS: "Be thankful for what you have"

1	2	3	4	5	6	7	8	9	10
Low				**Moderate**					**High**

14. SUPPORTIVE SYSTEM SKILLS: "Connect with family, friends and community"

1	2	3	4	5	6	7	8	9	10
Low				**Moderate**					**High**

15. LOVING SKILLS: "Do unto others as you would have them do unto you"

1	2	3	4	5	6	7	8	9	10
Low				**Moderate**					**High**

16. SPIRITUALITY SKILLS: Emuna "One's unconditional faith in G-d" (or higher power)

1	2	3	4	5	6	7	8	9	10
Low				**Moderate**					**High**

In this chapter, you have learned ten facts about your chronic pain. To review:

- Your chronic pain is not new. The intensity of it is.
- Your chronic pain is subjective. It's based on how you experience it.
- Your chronic pain is different than another person's pain. No two people will experience pain the same way.
- Your chronic pain is multi-dimensional. It may consist of your physical pain, your emotional pain, your pain from life stressors, your pain from negative thinking, and your pain from lack of fortitude.
- You may always have chronic pain. What may change is the intensity of it.
- Some of your coping strategies may be better than others. You can now determine which strategies aren't the most helpful to you.
- You must let go of "the way you were" before chronic pain. To hold on to wishing that your pain would disappear is to deny that your life has changed dramatically since having chronic pain.
- You may differ from others with chronic pain in your motivation to change how you are coping.
- Times are changing rapidly, and this impacts how you're dealing with your pain.
- You are free to choose the ways you use to lower your chronic pain. There are many strategies available to you to try out.

My intention in presenting these facts to you is to help you see your chronic pain as a "challenge" and an "opportunity" to grow and overcome it, rather than feeling despair. Since your pain is multi-dimensional, it is unrealistic for a medical specialist to simply say to you, "On a scale of one to five, what is your pain level?" You will share with your medical specialist your subjective level of physical pain. But, you may also have pain from your emotional states, pain from life stressors, pain from negative thinking or, pain from a lack of fortitude. To change your perception of your chronic pain in a positive way, I have showed you how to use five different scales that measure the multiple dimensions of your chronic pain. You've seen examples of how different people experienced their chronic pain and then measured it on each scale. In the next chapter, we'll explore a "case study" of someone who experiences chronic pain and has measured her pain levels on these five dimensions.

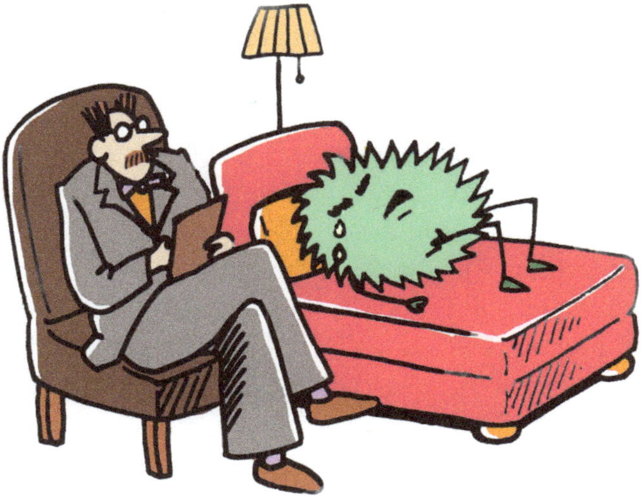

Doc! My whole family has been misunderstood!

Chapter 5: A Case Study

This chapter presents you with an opportunity to read a short "case study" of a woman named Joanne who experiences chronic pain, and has measured her pain levels on all five dimensions. After reading about Joanne's situation, you will see how she rated herself on all five scales, and I'll ask you to see if you can come up with ways to help her. Then you can compare your strategies with specific strategies I share with you in the subsequent chapters to help people like you and Joanne reduce your chronic pain.

Joanne is a 48-year-old married woman with two children who experiences heightened anxiety and severe chronic, physical pain in her left ankle following a recent fall on a piece of ice in her driveway. She is overweight and physically inactive much of the time, and was so even before the fall, except for driving her children to and from local activities. Two years ago, she had surgery on a tendon stretching from her right elbow to her right shoulder. She has finally obtained disability insurance for her constant pain and anxiety (which included ongoing panic attacks). Prior to obtaining disability, she had lost her full-time job as a veterinarian technician because of frequent absences due to both anxiety and pain.

After the recent fall, Joanne's husband, Mike, took her immediately to the hospital emergency room where an X-ray revealed that she had several ankle bone fragmentations. The ER staff recommended that she immediately see her medical team. In turn, her clinical nurse practitioner referred Joanne to an orthopedic surgeon who surgically inserted a plate with screws to stabilize her ankle. Joanne returned home two days later with crutches and a seven-day refillable prescription for Vicodin. After four weeks of home care (including nursing, physical and occupational therapy) she met again with her orthopedic surgeon. Another X-ray revealed that one of the stabilizing plate screws had loosened, but the surgeon didn't believe that would cause her any additional pain. He informed Joanne and Mike that he wouldn't remove the plate until the bones could solidify and she could increase her mobility through ongoing physical therapy. The surgeon further recommended that Joanne wean herself off the Vicodin and stick to taking NSAIDs like ibuprofen or naproxen, or use acetaminophen.

For the next three months, Joanne did little to improve her condition. She continued to feel much pain but secretly obtained opiates from an acquaintance. After home services stopped, Joanne scheduled physical therapy appointments but often canceled them at the last minute because she was in "too much pain." She did little to exercise or stretch and became more depressed while continuing to secretly take opiates, and spent much of her time lying in bed. At one point, her husband thought about taking her back to the ER because she had expressed some suicidal thoughts. When he discovered that Joanne was using street opiates, he made an emergency appointment with her primary care physician, who recommended a detoxification program. Joanne's physician further recommended that, once she was detoxed, she consider getting on methadone or Suboxone (buprenorphine), attend a weekly clinic, then meet with the team's health psychologist to address where she was in her motivation to change.

Joanne did these things and saw the health psychologist the following week. He listened attentively and without judgment to Joanne's concerns and how she presently dealt with her pain. He expressed empathy for how she had been enduring pain, even before her fall.

The health psychologist obtained Joanne's permission to collaborate with Mike to make sure Joanne weaned herself off the opiates over time. She also attended an outpatient drug treatment program for at least two weeks in addition to her medication clinic. She further agreed to see the health psychologist in the late afternoons.

The health psychologist then questioned Joanne, without judgment, and without giving advice, about the ways she was choosing to cope with her pain. He wondered how her choices had been both helpful and harmful for reducing pain. Together, they did a cost-benefit analysis of her present methods, including the use of opiates, being overweight, keeping physical therapy appointments inconsistently, and being anxious and idle. The health psychologist emphasized the need for Joanne to consider both the short-term and long-term consequences of her choices. By doing this, Joanne realized that most of her present strategies for reducing pain were not effective, especially her reliance on opiates. She acknowledged that she had to let go of these choices but the real issue for her was that she couldn't let go of thinking about how happy she had been before the onset of her chronic pain.

During the next few sessions, the health psychologist helped Joanne mourn how she was in the past prior to having severe pain. Together, they worked through each grief stage until Joanne could come to terms with accepting that she might always have pain, but it didn't have to be so intolerable.

Next, the health psychologist explained to Joanne how chronic pain is multi-dimensional, that it is subjective (meaning each person's experience of pain is different), and that pain is a metaphor for all kinds of pain, including one's emotional states, life stressors, negative thinking, and the degree to which one uses one's strengths to deal with chronic pain. He told Joanne that she could reframe her chronic pain as a challenge and as an opportunity to test her strengths in dealing with life changes.

He brought out the Chronic Pain Scales, reviewed the instructions for each one, including how to score them, then explained that the overall goal was to do whatever it took to reduce the negative pain scale ratings to between 1 and 3 and increase the positive scale ratings to between 7 and 10, weekly over time. He offered her the same strategies to reduce chronic pain that are provided in the next few chapters, and explained that "one size doesn't fit all." What would work for her would be different from what worked for other people who have chronic pain. The strategies that people choose need to be acted upon on a trial basis. If one or some didn't work, then Joanne should try others.

The health psychologist told Joanne that it would be helpful if she could review the strategies at home with Mike, then choose the ones she planned to use. He asked if she could complete the five scales at least twice during the week, then meet again the following week to see if they noticed any patterns. Joanne agreed to complete the scales at home with her husband's assistance and to bring them back to the health psychologist to assess at periodic check-ins every few weeks after the next week's appointment.

Here are the initial scales that Joanna completed:

PHYSICAL PAIN SCALE

NAME: JOANNE DATE: 6/8/17

Please rate your physical pain during the day, per hour, on a scale from 1-10. Please describe what you are doing, the location of the pain, whether it is constant or comes and goes and, what the pain is like using the adjectives on the next page.

TIME: 12:00 PM — LEFT ANKLE — 1 2 3 4 (5) 6 7 8 9 10
Low Pain / Moderate Pain / Intense Pain

JUST GOT HOME, WALKED UPSTAIRS AND AROUND HOUSE, PAIN IS CONSTANT, IT'S A SHARP ACHING PAIN, TOOK 800MGS IBUPROFEN

TIME: 2:12 PM — LEFT ANKLE — 1 2 3 (4) 5 6 7 8 9 10
Low Pain / Moderate Pain / Intense Pain

JUST DID DISHES AND MADE A TUNA SANDWICH FOR MYSELF PAIN IS CONSTANT AND ITS STILL FLICKERING WITH EACH STEP

TIME: 3:20PM — LEFT ANKLE + ACHILLES TENDON — 1 2 3 4 (5) 6 7 8 9 10
Low Pain / Moderate Pain / Intense Pain

JUST GOT BACK FROM DROPPING DAUGHTER OFF AT WORK. AND CLIMBING STAIRS. PAIN IS SHARP ACHING

TIME: 4:30PM — LEFT ANKLE, RIGHT ELBOW — 1 2 3 (4) 5 6 7 8 9 10
Low Pain / Moderate Pain / Intense Pain

BEEN LAYING DOWN WATCHING TV, PAIN EASED A LITTLE, TO A DULL ACHE, RIGHT ELBOW STARTING TO ACHE (HAD TENNIS ELBOW SURGERY 2 YRS AGO, STILL BOTHERS ME)

TIME: 5:20PM — 1 2 3 4 (5) 6 7 8 9 10
Low Pain / Moderate Pain / Intense Pain

WENT TO GET AC IN MY CAR CHARGED, ANKLE FEELING SORER NOW A SHARP ACHING ALL AROUND MY ANKLE.

LEFT ANKLE

TIME: 6:40 PM 1 2 3 4 5 (6) 7 8 9 10
Low Pain Moderate Pain Intense Pain

ATE HALF OF A DRY STEAK BOMB FOR SUPPER, SETTLING DOWN FOR THE NIGHT, TINGLING AND ACHING PAIN TOOK 800 MGS OF IBUPROFEN

LEFT ANKLE + LEG

TIME: 7:45 1 2 3 4 5 (6) 7 8 9 10
Low Pain Moderate Pain Intense Pain

WATCHING 3RD SEASON OF PRISON BREAK, OUTER LEFT ANKLE VERY SORE, RADIATING UP MY LEG, IBUPROFEN NOT AS HELPFUL AS IT WAS EARLIER

LEFT ANKLE

TIME: 8:55 1 2 3 4 5 (6) 7 8 9 10
Low Pain Moderate Pain Intense Pain

WATCHING TV, HAVE LEFT FOOT UP ON 3 PILLOWS, PAIN IS achin around ankle

Some words that can help you describe the way your painfeels. Is it ___

Aching?	Cramping?	Taut?	Binding?	Gnawing?
Freezing?	Unbearable?	Heavy?	Hot or burning?	Nagging?
Numb?	(Sharp?)	Shooting?	Squeezing?	Cold?
Sickening?	Splitting?	Tight?	Dreadful?	Stabbing?
Punishing or cruel?	Cool?	Bolts?	Tender?	Throbbing?
Agonizing?	Excruciating?	Tiring?	Distressing?	Stiffness?
Pulling?	Flickering?	Pricking?	Pinching?	Stabbing?
Mild?	Intense?	Pulsating?	Intermittent?	Scalding?
Exhausting?	Sore?	Sharp?	Terrifying?	Killing?
Beating?	Jumping?	Miserable?	Piercing?	Drilling?
Cutting?	Tearing?	Nauseating?	Constant?	Stinging?
Electrical?	Pounding?	Tugging?	Splitting?	Knot-like?
Horrible?	Smarting?	Pins/Needles?	(Radiating?)	Waving?
Rasping?	Annoying?	~~Quivering?~~	Icthy?	Suffocating?
Spreading?	(Dull?)	(Tingling?)	Grueling?	Drawing?

PHYSICAL PAIN SCALE

Please rate your physical pain for **2 days during the morning,afternoon, and evening** on a scale from 1-10. Please describe what you are doing, the location of the pain, whether it is constant or comes and goes and, what the pain is like using the adjectives on the next page.

DATE: 6/10/17

Morning Time: 8 AM

1 2 3 4 5 6 7 8 9 10
Low Pain · Moderate Pain · Intense Pain

JUST GOT UP, LESS WHEN RELAXED FROM EVENING
MILD IN LEFT ANKLE

Afternoon Time: 1 PM

1 2 3 4 5 6 7 8 9 10
Low Pain · Moderate Pain · Intense Pain

WALKING WITH A FRIEND, HAD TO STOP A LOT PAIN
IN LEFT ANKLE PIERCING SHARP

Evening Time: 8PM

1 2 3 4 5 6 7 8 9 10
Low Pain · Moderate Pain · Intense Pain

STILL IN PAIN FROM DOING DISHES, FATIGUE RIGHT
ELBOW. STINGING, DULL ACHE, LEFT ANKLE SHARP

DATE: 6/12/17

Morning Time: 7:30AM

1 2 3 4 5 6 7 8 9 10
Low Pain · Moderate Pain · Intense Pain

LESS PAIN, SLEEP HELPS AS DOES NOT MOVING
DULL, NUMB

Afternoon Time: 11:30 AM

1 2 3 4 5 6 7 (8) 9 ~~10~~
Low Pain Moderate Pain (Intense Pain)

REALLY HURTS, TRIED TO WALK FOR A MILE. LEFT ANKLE SHARP, STINGING, ELBOW OK WHEN DON'T LIFT ANYTHING

Evening Time: 8:00 PM

1 2 ~~3~~ 4 5 6 (7) 8 9 10
Low Pain Moderate Pain Intense Pain

LEG & ANKLE PAIN IS ~~INTENSE~~ CONSTANT, TRY TO DO SOME HOUSEWORK, RIGHT ELBOW ALSO STABBING FROM USING UTENSILS.

Some words that can help you describe the way your painfeels. Is it ___

Aching?	Cramping?	Taut?	Binding?	Gnawing?
Freezing?	Unbearable?	Heavy?	Hot or burning?	Nagging?
Numb?	Sharp?	Shooting?	Squeezing?	Cold?
Sickening?	Splitting?	Tight?	Dreadful?	Stabbing?
Punishing or cruel?	Cool?	Bolts?	Tender?	Throbbing?
Agonizing?	Excruciating?	Tiring?	Distressing?	Stiffness?
Pulling?	Flickering?	Pricking?	Pinching?	Stabbing?
Mild?	Intense?	Pulsating?	Intermittent?	Scalding?
Exhausting?	Sore?	Sharp?	Terrifying?	Killing?
Beating?	Jumping?	Miserable?	Piercing?	Drilling?
Cutting?	Tearing?	Nauseating?	Constant?	Stinging?
Electrical?	Pounding?	Tugging?	Splitting?	Knot-like?
Horrible?	Smarting?	Pins/Needles?	Radiating?	Waving?
Rasping?	Annoying?	Quivering?	Icthy?	Suffocating?
Spreading?	Dull?	Tingling?	Grueling?	Drawing?

LIFE STRESS PAIN SCALE

Please review your present experiences of stress below and rate on a scale of 1-10 the degree to which you believe each stress below impacts your pain.

NAME: JOANNE **DATE:** 6/8/17

- [ ] Housing
- [ ] Engagement
- [ ] Pregnancy
- [x] Teenagers
- [ ] In-laws
- [ ] Hobbies
- [ ] Single
- [ ] Hours at Work
- [x] Finances
- [ ] Rape
- [ ] Natural Catastrophe
- [ ] Caring for Elder(s)
- [ ] Legal Issues
- [x] Insurance Concerns
- [ ] Workman's Compensation
- [ ] Experiencing/ Witnessing/Hearing About Trama
- [ ] Education
- [x] Relationships
- [ ] Childbirth
- [ ] Parents
- [ ] Friendships
- [ ] Affair(s)
- [ ] Post-Marital Conflict
- [ ] Increased Work Responsibilities
- [ ] Wills/Estates
- [ ] Death of Loved One
- [ ] Lack of Assertiveness
- [ ] Substance Use/ Abuse
- [x] Medical Issues
- [ ] Getting/ Not Getting Disability Insurance
- [ ] Retirement
- [ ] Isolation
- [x] Marital Problems
- [ ] Children's Illness
- [ ] Role Functions
- [ ] Social Life
- [ ] Separation
- [ ] Single Parenting
- [ ] Multi-Tasking Demands
- [x] Aging
- [ ] Grandparenting
- [ ] Religious Affiliation
- [ ] Other Addictions (Porn, Internet, Gambling, etc)
- [ ] Hospitalization(s)
- [ ] Listening to or Watching News
- [ ] Courting
- [ ] Infertility
- [ ] Raising Children
- [ ] Siblings
- [ ] Lack of Exercise
- [ ] Divorce
- [ ] Balancing Parenting and work
- [ ] Career Issues/ Dissatisfaction
- [ ] War
- [ ] Unemployment
- [ ] Verbal or Physical Abuse
- [ ] Getting into an Accident (with/without) injuries
- [x] Surgery(ies)
- [ ] Politics
- [x] Other: dependency on prescribed Medications

Please indicate the overall (average) rating of present stress that impacts your pain.

1	2	3	4	5	(6)	7	8	9	10
Not a problem				Somewhat of a problem			A very large problem		

and its -

Impact on Family (1-10)	Impact on Work (1-10)	Impact on Social Life (1-10)
9	10	8

EMOTIONAL PAIN SCALE

NAME: JOANNE **DATE:** 6/8/17

Please review your present experiences of the emotional conditions noted below and rate on a scale of 1-10 the degree to which you believe each one has an impact on your level of pain.

If you have a significant other person in your life please consider asking him/her to help you rate this scale.

(1 = I do not believe this to be true) to (10 = I believe this to be true)

Note: Happiness Scale is scored differnetly than the other three scales-the higher the score, the better the rating.

1. DEPRESSION:

1 2 3 4 5 6 (7) 8 9 10

Low (low-sad-hurt) **Moderate** (unhappy-aggrieved-dejected) **Severe** (depressed-miserable-despondent)

2. ANXIETY:

1 2 3 4 5 6 7 (8) 9 10

Low (concerned-uncomfortable-bothered) **Moderate** (worried-upset-troubled) **Severe** (frightened-overwhelmed-panicky)

3. ANGER:

1 (2) 3 4 5 6 7 8 9 `10

Low (annoyed-hurt-disappointed) **Moderate** (frustrated-upset-mad) **Severe** (furious-enraged-incensed)

4. HAPPINESS:

1 (2) 3 4 5 6 7 8 9 10

Low (glad-comfortable-content) **Moderate** (cheerful-pleased-happy) **Severe** (blissful-exhilarated-ecstatic)

COGNITIVE APPRAISAL OF PAIN SCALE

NAME: JOANNE **DATE:** 6/8/17

Please these different cognitive appraials and rate on a scale of 1-10 the degree to which you believe each appraisal to be true for you.

If you have a significant other person in your life please consider asking him/her to help you rate this scale.

(1 = I do not believe this to be true) to (10 = I believe this to be true)

1. **ALL OR NOTHING THINKING (Dichotomous Thinking):**
   You view most situations as two distinct categories (always vs. never, perfect vs. terrible)
   "I can't work because I always have pain." " I never feel good."
   1 2 3 4 5 6 7 8 (9) 10
   A little Some A Lot

2. **OVER GENERALIZATION:**
   You make global negative conclusions that go well beyond the one situation.
   "I can't do what I used to do because I can't bike." "I won't be able to do anything because I can't walk long distances."
   1 2 3 4 5 6 7 8 9 (10)
   A little Some A Lot

3. **MENTAL FILTERING:**
   You pay more attention to a single detail instead of seeing the whole picture.
   "My pain means that I'm inadequate."
   1 2 3 4 5 6 7 8 (9) 10
   A little Some A Lot

4. **DISQUALIFYING THE POSITIVE:**
   You tell yourself that positive experiences don't count.
   "I was able to cook one meal last night but one night out of twenty doesn't mean much."
   1 2 3 4 5 6 7 8 9 (10)
   A little Some A Lot

5. **JUMPING TO CONCLUSIONS - FUTURISTIC THINKING:**
   You focus on the the future and predict it negatively without considering other possibilities.
   "Oh no! Here comes the pain again. I'll definitely wind up in the emergency room."
   1 2 3 4 5 6 (7) 8 9 10
   A little Some A Lot

6. **CATASTROPHIZING - MAGNIFICATION:**
   You exaggerate the importance of things and minimize the positive, you think of the worst versus the best case scenario. You make a mountain out of a molehill.
   "My pain will be totally unbearable."
   1 2 3 4 5 6 7 (8) 9 10
   A little Some A Lot

8. **SELF-MONITORING SKILLS:** "Think before you act"

1 2 3 4 5 6 7 8 9 10
Low Moderate High

9. **COGNITIVE FLEXIBILITY SKILLS:** "Go with the flow"

1 2 3 4 5 6 7 8 9 10
Low Moderate High

10. **OPTIMISM SKILLS:** "Hope for the future"

1 2 3 4 5 6 7 8 9 10
Low Moderate High

11. **HUMOR SKILLS:** "Laugh and the whole world laughs with you"

1 2 3 4 5 6 7 8 9 10
Low Moderate High

12. **RESILIENCY SKILLS:** "You can bounce back"

1 2 3 4 5 6 7 8 9 10
Low Moderate High

13. **GRATITUDE SKILLS:** "Be thankful for what you have"

1 2 3 4 5 6 7 8 9 10
Low Moderate High

14. **SUPPORTIVE SYSTEM SKILLS:** "Connect with family, friends and community"

1 2 3 4 5 6 7 8 9 10
Low Moderate High

15. **LOVING SKILLS:** "Do unto others as you would have them do unto you"

1 2 3 4 5 6 7 8 9 10
Low Moderate High

16. **SPIRITUALITY SKILLS:** Emuna "One's unconditional faith in G-d" (or higher power)

1 2 3 4 5 6 7 8 9 10
Low Moderate High

FORTITUDE SCALE

NAME: Joanne **DATE:** 6/8/17

Please review your present experiences of the conditions noted below and rate on a scale of 1-10 the degree to which you believe each condition has an impact on your level of pain.

Note: The higher the rating, the stronger the belief.

If you have a significant other person in your life please consider asking him/her to help you rate this scale.
(1 = I do not believe this to be true to (10 = I believe this to be true)

1. **COPING SKILLS:** "You can handle it"
   1 2 (3) 4 5 6 7 8 9 10
   Low **Moderate** **High**

2. **SELF-ESTEEM:** "Feel good about yourself"
   Balance between

   A. SELF-CARE SKILLS "You can handle it"
   1 (2) 3 4 5 6 7 8 9 10
   Low **Moderate** **High**

   And B.. SELF-EFFICACY SKILLS "Accomplish things"
   1 (2) 3 4 5 6 7 8 9 10
   Low **Moderate** **High**

3. **ASSSERIVENESS SKILLS:** "Stand up for your rights"
   1 2 3 (4) 5 6 7 8 9 10
   Low **Moderate** **High**

4. **EXERCISE SKILLS:** "Just do it!"
   1 (2) 3 4 5 6 7 8 9 10
   Low **Moderate** **High**

5. **DISTRACTION SKILLS:** "Take the time to smell the roses"
   1 (2) 3 4 5 6 7 8 9 10
   Low **Moderate** **High**

6. **MINFULNESS SKILLS:** "Be here now!"
   1 2 (3) 4 5 6 7 8 9 10
   Low **Moderate** **High**

7. **PROBLEM SOLVING SKILLS:** "What is your problem?""What are some of your plans?" "What is the best plan?"" Act on your plan""How did you do?"
   1 2 3 4 (5) 6 7 8 9 10
   Low **Moderate** **High**

8. **SELF-MONITORING SKILLS:** "Think before you act"

1	2	3	4	5	6	7	8	9	10
Low				Moderate					High

9. **COGNITIVE FLEXIBILITY SKILLS:** "Go with the flow"

1	2	3	4	5	6	7	8	9	10
Low				Moderate					High

10. **OPTIMISM SKILLS:** "Hope for the future"

1	2	3	4	5	6	7	8	9	10
Low				Moderate					High

11. **HUMOR SKILLS:** "Laugh and the whole world laughs with you"

1	2	3	4	5	6	7	8	9	10
Low				Moderate					High

12. **RESILIENCY SKILLS:** "You can bounce back"

1	2	3	4	5	6	7	8	9	10
Low				Moderate					High

13. **GRATITUDE SKILLS:** "Be thankful for what you have"

1	2	3	4	5	6	7	8	9	10
Low				Moderate					High

14. **SUPPORTIVE SYSTEM SKILLS:** "Connect with family, friends and community"

1	2	3	4	5	6	7	8	9	10
Low				Moderate					High

15. **LOVING SKILLS:** "Do unto others as you would have them do unto you"

1	2	3	4	5	6	7	8	9	10
Low				Moderate					High

16. **SPIRITUALITY SKILLS:** Emuna "One's unconditional faith in G-d" (or higher power)

1	2	3	4	5	6	7	8	9	10
Low				Moderate					High

Upon meeting with Joanne again in a week's time, the health psychologist first acknowledged how well she had been able to get around and do multiple daily tasks and that most of her pain rating levels between 4 and 6 weren't so bad. He further noticed that she had sharp, dull or aching pain and that it was more constant than variable. Sometimes, the pain radiated through her leg. Together, they thought that it might be helpful to first re-review this concern with her primary care physician or clinical nurse practitioner to see if she needed a referral to another specialist, such as a neurologist, a medical pain specialist like an anesthesiologist for possible injections, or perhaps a physical therapist or chiropractor. At least for now, the health psychologist recommended taking short breaks to ease the pain rather than wait to lie down at night where she rated the pain levels as a 3.

Joanne experienced severe depression and anxiety but had limited anger and irritability. She internalized her symptoms, which probably aggravated her pain condition. Clearly, Joanne wasn't a very happy person at this time, given her low rating scale of 3 on the Happiness Scale.

The health psychologist pointed out how Joanne had multiple negative thoughts that contributed immensely to her chronic pain. She rated all the appraisals on the Cognitive Appraisal of Pain Scale high except for "Personalization," meaning she didn't necessarily blame herself excessively for her pain, although she rated "Labeling" as high. This implied that the extent of her high negative ratings on this scale contributed to Joanne having an overall negative schema or belief about herself as being "stupid" or "not good enough."

Joanne had multiple life stressors contributing to her pain. Her high ratings of life stress impacting on work, family and relationships indicated her stressors were strong influences on how she experienced chronic pain.

Of the most concern were Joanne's low scale ratings for many areas of strength needed to reduce chronic pain. The only high rating on her Fortitude Scale was in her capacity to experience the humorous aspects of situations. While humor is a positive strength, several other areas could be more easily strengthened than others, like trying to be grateful and loving. Still, Joanne needed much help in developing critical skills like self-esteem, the capacity to cope, being resilient, optimistic and appreciative of the positive aspects of life.

You Try It!

If you were Joanne, what specific goals would you want to identify to help lower the negative rating scales to 1-3 and increase the positive ones to 7-10 over time? Try to think of five goals for each of the five scales, and make them as realistic and as specific as possible. You may want to divide goals into sub-goals, if necessary.

Physical Goals

1. ______________________________

2. ______________________________

3. ______________________________

4. ______________________________

5. ______________________________

Emotional Goals

1. ______________________________

2. ______________________________

3. ______________________________

4. ______________________________

5. ______________________________

Life Stressor Goals

1. ______________________________

2. ______________________________

3. ______________________________

4. ______________________________

5. ______________________________

Negative Thinking Goals

1. ______________________________

2. ______________________________

3. ______________________________

4. ______________________________

5. ______________________________

Fortitude Goals

1. ______________________________

2. ______________________________

3. ______________________________

4. ______________________________

5. ______________________________

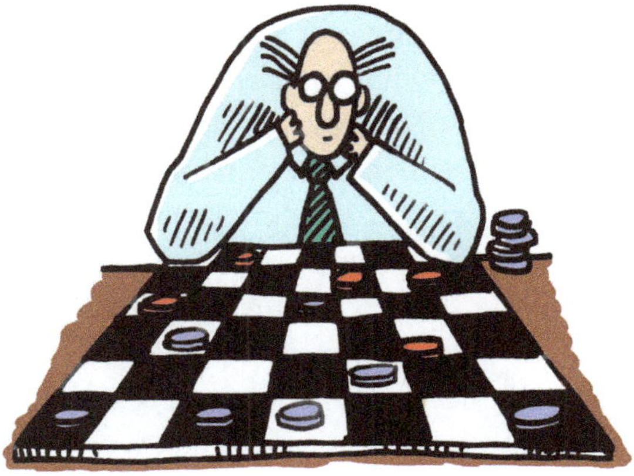

Ponder your next move carefully.

Chapter 6: Strategies to Reduce Chronic Pain

Now that you have read Joanne's story (in the previous chapter) and have written down suggested goals for her, I want you to read the specific strategies I identify in the next few chapters, and determine which strategies would be best for Joanne, and for you!

There are many ways to explore how to reduce your physical pain. You can search the internet, download applications, watch YouTube videos, listen to podcasts or read blogs or books. While you can do a lot of searching, you may find that the strategies below are a great place to start. You will benefit from what I have learned to try first to reduce your chronic pain. Review these, and then read about specific strategies you may want to try for each pain scale.

There are two major stages to pain reduction. The first is pain loss or doing whatever it takes to reduce pain. The second is pain maintenance or preventing relapses of pain flare-ups over time. Relapse prevention is just as important as pain reduction. Your intention should be to keep your pain to minimal levels as best as you can. This would be defined as ratings of 1-4 for negative scaled items on the Physical Pain Scale, the Life Stressor Pain Scale, the Emotional Scale, and the Cognitive Appraisal of Pain Scale, and ratings of 7-10 for positive scaled items on the Emotional and Fortitude Scales. Know your specific triggers that can increase pain flare-ups, especially those triggers that can increase negative thoughts. Of course, there are situations you can control and those that you can't control, such as some major life stressors.

In all areas of behavior change -- whether it be reducing your pain, your weight, your diabetes, your cholesterol, or your abuse of alcohol, opiates, tobacco, or cannabis beyond what has been prescribed for medical purposes -- the most critical elements of success are your having sufficient support systems in place and knowing which of your triggers can induce relapse.

In fact, relapse prevention is just as important as pain reduction. The goal is to reduce and maintain your negative pain scale ratings, improve your positive ones, and then sustain them, keeping the rating levels steady over time.

People's inability to maintain behavior change over time is why most plans often fail. For example, many people go on a diet, then regain their lost weight. Why? Because they don't have maintenance strategies in place to keep their weight within a reasonable range over time. The same is often true when it comes to chronic pain reduction and painless maintenance. You must have strategies and support in place to succeed!

Remember, there is a difference between controlling your pain and having no pain. You may always have pain, when you consider that physical pain is impacted by multiple factors, like your emotions, life stressors, negative thoughts and fortitude, or lack thereof.

While it is critical to establish and maintain a support system, no one else can truly appreciate the level of pain that you experience, not even your closest loved ones. Still, you must do everything you can to involve them in your Pain Management Lifestyle. Educate them about what your pain is like, when you have it, and what you are doing to reduce it. It may be helpful to have them attend a session with your pain management clinician or health psychologist so they can learn what you are going through and how you are trying to overcome these experiences by committing to certain strategies. Have them understand that you are grieving the loss of how you once were before you had the high pain intensity. Ask them to be understanding if you "lose it" once in a while, as it is common for those with pain to experience high levels of anxiety, anger or depression.

Helpful Strategies to Maintain Your Pain Reduction Over Time

Here's a list of seven strategies to use in your own Pain Management Lifestyle as you focus on reducing your pain to the degree that you can and learn the next ways for you to manage the pain that remains.

1. Use the five pain scales provided in this book to self-monitor how you are doing on a weekly basis. Note what needs to be reduced (to a level between 1 and 4) and what needs to improve (to a level between 7 and 10), then plan and act on ways to do so over time. Remember that your pain scale results are snapshots of what your experience is at that moment in time. Make copies of the scales in Chapters 7 through to 11 or email the author at drgeorgepainless@gmail.com and complete them at least once weekly to see how you are doing.

2. Know what your high-scoring negative thoughts tend to be, especially those that trigger emotional pain (anxiety, depression and anger).

3. Use your head! That is, improve the use of your prefrontal cortex, especially the specific executive functions of self-monitoring (catching yourself generating negative thoughts) and practicing sufficient fortitude skills, cognitive flexibility (shifting and adjusting when upsets or changes occur), and healthy problem-solving.

4. Have a support system in place. Review your ongoing progress regularly with your pain management team. This includes your pain management clinician (health psychologist), your primary care physician and clinical nurse practitioner. The clinician should be a medical specialist like a physician's assistant, a licensed psychologist, or a social worker with particular experience and training in pain management. Join a support group and take advantage of websites and social media groups and learn from other people trying to reduce chronic pain.

5. Make sure your caretaker(s) (whether they are spouses, cohabiters, family members or best friends) obtain enough support through good self-care practices. You don't want to burn them out! The significant others in your life need support as well, and need to take care of themselves. You don't want to criticize, alienate or lose them. Rather, you should respect that they need refueling through their own support systems and taking the time to engage in their preferred self-care activities. Keep them regularly apprised of how

you are doing. They should meet periodically with your pain management team to stay informed and provide the team with input that helps them collaborate effectively with you to tailor pain reduction and maintenance strategies to your needs.

6. Go slowly! Have realistic expectations and measure them through sub-goals, rather than anticipating a dramatic change from one level of the pain scales to another. If you become frustrated, it is probably due to high self-standards or not fully letting go of what you were formerly capable of doing before chronic pain entered your life.

7. Maintain the strategies that you and your pain management team have chosen and continue to monitor how they are helping or not helping you to reduce your negative pain scale ratings and improve your positive ones. Change or modify them if they are not effective. One size doesn't fit all!

Now that we've taken a broad overview of pain management strategies, let's turn next to specific ways to reduce pain in each of the five areas we've discussed in the book (physical, life stressors, emotional, negative thoughts, and fortitude).

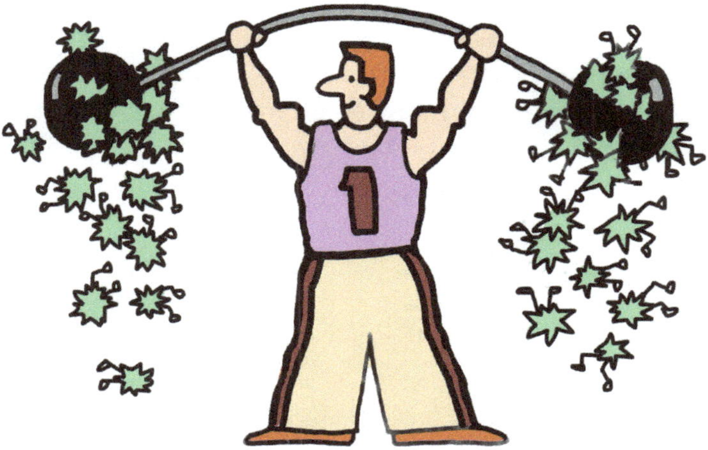

You are your own SUPER person.

Chapter 7: Physical Ways to Reduce Your Pain

The recommendations I include in this chapter are the ones I have found the most helpful, both as a professional who has worked with people like you who have experienced chronic pain and as someone who personally has had chronic pain. It's important to realize that a majority of the medical community will focus on physical recommendations, like the ones in this chapter, rather than the recommendations suggested in the next few chapters that focus on other critical ways to reduce your pain.

1. Don't stay in bed! It's very easy to hunker down, put the covers over your body and rest your head on a soft pillow to withdraw from the reality of having to get up and face another day of chronic pain. Just as tempting is the notion of sitting in a chair all day watching TV and eating to your hearts' content while becoming more depressed or anxious. Yes, these activities may feel good and comfy, and it's your choice! But it's not the best choice, either in the short or the long term. You'll experience greater stiffness, muscle atrophy and pain from discs that fill with fluid while lying down and hurt when you get up. Staying in bed will cause the significant others in your life to become concerned or even frustrated and angry. Avoidance and withdrawal are coping techniques but they're not the best way to reduce chronic pain.

2. Get better sleep. Do you sleep poorly? Have a hard time getting to sleep? Do you get up frequently? Do you feel still tired in the morning? Is it difficult for you to get between seven and nine hours of sleep and feel rested in the morning? These problems can be caused by simple things like eating or using electronic devices too close to bedtime, or drinking too much caffeine. Poor sleep can correlate highly with stress, anxiety, and depression, or a combination of these factors.
   If good sleep is a problem, then tell your medical team so they can help you determine what's going on. Reviewing your different scale ratings will help you identify what may be affecting your sleep. In some instances, sleep problems may be caused by other medical problems or a combination of factors. For example, being overweight may be related to having sleep apnea; if that's possible for you, then request a sleep study. If you discover that you have even moderate sleep apnea, then get and use the newest versions of the CPAP machine. As awkward as it may feel, you will notice an incredible difference not only in falling asleep but not getting up all the time even to urinate and you'll cut out the snoring and will feel incredibly rested in the morning. You will even be able to sleep again in the same bed with your spouse or significant other!

3. How comfortable is your bed? Too hard? Too soft? Too small? I found that a hard bed was giving me incredible muscle spasms in the morning. Make sure your bed feels comfortable and provides for less pain while you sleep and when you wake up.

4. Develop a morning ritual. When you get up in the morning, meditate, do a mindfulness exercise, or pray for at least 10 minutes. Second, identify five things or people to whom you are forever grateful. Keep a sense of perspective – some days it may simply include the fact that you are still alive and breathing or that your situation could be worse! Third, listen to some relaxing or inspiring music as you get out of bed. It will soothe your soul. Fourth, massage out any stiffness in your muscles by using a foam roller. It's like having your own masseuse. Fifth, stretch, doing only those warm-up stretches before you do any aerobic exercise (fast walking, swimming, biking) and standing-still stretches after you do any aerobic exercise that are recommended by your medical specialists. Certain stretches

before and after you exercise aerobically can do more harm than good, depending on your physical ailments. Discuss the use of an elastic exercise band for a variety of stretches. It's a wonderful tool for improving flexibility and strength.

5. See your specialists. Be assertive in making sure you meet with whichever specialist is necessary to clarify the cause of any clear physical condition that could be exacerbating your pain. Your pain management team should be the primary source to determine what medical tests need to be done and what specialists you should be authorized to see.

6. Seek multiple solutions. There is no single solution and no easy way to reduce pain. Physical pain can come simply from poor posture and movement patterns. Core strengthening and keeping to extension or inflexion movements that reduce pain, not aggravate it, is critical. Again, it is best to have a full-range workup to determine which postures or movements cause you the most pain, then identify specific exercises that will be most helpful.

7. Know what's enough. There is a distinction between "doing too much" and "doing too little" to obtain medical evidence that supports a clear physical cause for your pain that may need specific treatment or surgery in some cases. What is "enough" should be based on a realistic appraisal in collaboration with your pain management team, rather than getting caught up in all-or-nothing thinking (known as a negative cognitive appraisal), or trying to meet unrealistic standards. It's always more of a relief to find a clear physical cause for your chronic pain, but remember that pain is subjective, multi-dimensional and influenced by other factors that increase pain. These other factors include co-existing depression, anxiety, anger, lack of happiness, life stressors, negative thoughts and lack of fortitude. If you don't consider these additional factors on an ongoing basis, then you'll be constantly searching for a physical cause.

8. Maintain multiple strategies that you and your pain management team have chosen. Continue to monitor how they are helping or not helping you to reduce your negative pain scale ratings and improve the positive ones. Change them if they are not helping. One size doesn't fit all!

9. Do not rely on opiates as a major way to reduce chronic pain! While some people need to be on opiates for some time, be aware that pain management teams are reducing or eliminating opiate prescriptions due to the exponential increase of deaths from opiate overdoses. Even those anesthesiologists who were trained in pain management, and do trigger point injections, nerve blockers, neural ablations (nerve burning) and insert Transdermal Electronic Nerve Stimulators (internal TENS units) are veering away from prescribing opiates. There are other medicines that can help with pain. These include NSAIDS (like aspirin, ibuprofen and naproxen), acetaminophen, serotonin norepinephrine reuptake inhibitors (SNRIs), and some older Tricyclic Antidepressants (TCAs). It is always best to consider multiple pain reduction strategies that may possibly include medications, rather than depending solely on medications.

10. Build your team support network. When you are in the preparation stage of change, consider the importance of building your support network. Strongly consider the benefits of remaining engaged as long as you can in physical ways to increase strength and mobility. This usually means consistent meetings with a specialist who is well trained and experienced in the physical conditions of the body. If you decide to see a trainer, make sure they're knowledgeable about neuromuscular structure and that they collaborate with someone from your medical team.

11. Understand your X-ray and MRI reports and how the results impact your choice of the best ways to reduce your chronic pain. Collaborate with your pain management team to hear their perspectives and conclusions from reviewing these reports.

12. Maintain a healthy weight range. Obesity is a major cause of pain in the whole body and has become a major epidemic in the US. If you are overweight, you are at further risk for sleep apnea, diabetes, and high cholesterol and triglyceride levels. See a nutritionist on a regular basis to establish and maintain a healthy eating plan.

13. Eat nutritiously. Lose weight and maintain your weight within a healthy weight range. Watch your calorie intake daily and avoid

ingesting too many synthetic sugars and artificial sweeteners. Eat more fish and chicken and less meat. Include more vegetables and natural sweeteners like fruits in your diet. Avoid using saturated fats and pay attention to food labels. Stay away from high-calorie sweets and snacks. Instead, eat natural snacks like carrot sticks, celery, and nuts. Even air-popped popcorn is a good choice. Make an appointment with a nutritionist to determine what should be included in your meal plan, then meet on a regular basis to monitor your food intake.

14. No smoking or overeating! Do not turn to cigarette smoking or overeating as an alternative to losing and maintaining weight. That's simply exchanging one bad habit for another.

15. Walk! Walk! Walk! Even if it's just for a block or two at a time, followed by a rest. Even if you need a cane or a walker. Then walk again. Walking may seem too boring if you were formerly quite the athlete, but it's the best exercise for you. Set realistic sub-goals in walking. Walk a few blocks, then a quarter of a mile, then a half-mile, and build up the distance you can handle over time. If you have access to a pool year-round, then you can do your walking in the water. Using foam bar-bells or waterproof ankle weights when walking in water can help to strengthen your muscles.

16. Choose the right footwear. Make sure you're wearing comfortable walking or running shoes with excellent support, "bounce," and comfort. If you're not sure about what shoes to purchase, then consider seeing a podiatrist to assess your feet, gait and posture. You may need a specific type of shoe or an orthotic sole to insert in whatever shoe you wear.

17. Establish an exercise routine. Develop a daily structure for building endurance, improving posture, stretching, muscle strengthening and whatever exercises your pain management team has suggested based on their assessment of your individual condition. Getting into a routine is best because you'll feel more hopeful and you'll see positive results, especially if you establish

18. Alternate between moist heat and ice. Find the best fit for your physical pain.

19. Use a rubber exercise band to do stretching and muscle strengthening. I have found this simple tool to be so useful in so many ways, and you will too.

20. Listen to music as you do your daily physical routines. Music soothes the soul and provides much inspiration to help you remain persistent and hopeful.

21. Drink water! Drink at least eight (8) fluid ounces of water daily. Drinking enough water will reduce muscle spasms.

22. Review your physical pain rating scales on a weekly basis to spot particular patterns and identify what you are doing that works to reduce physical pain levels.

23. Set new goals. If you are finding your sub-goals are too difficult to achieve, then divide them into further sub-goals. The key is to not give up hope simply because you're frustrated that you can't do what you'd like to be doing. Lower your standards if needed, based on your body's signals.

I hope that these strategies to reduce your physical pain are as helpful to you as they've been to me. Most of the strategies are based on my professional experience in working with people just like you. Others are based on my personal experiences, having had chronic pain since that traumatic day in August 2008. Remember! What works for you to reduce your physical pain will be different from other people who experience chronic pain.

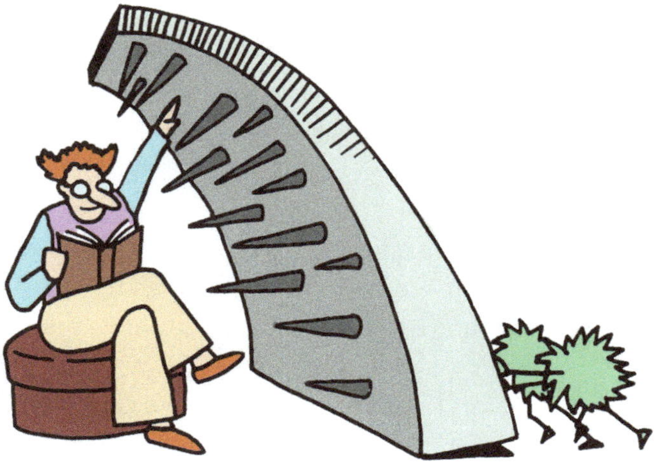

Try not to sweat the little things.

Chapter 8: Ways to Reduce Your Pain from Life Stressors

As we've emphasized throughout the book, chronic pain is not just physical – it can be influenced by life stressors. Some of the ways to reduce your life stressors may be more difficult than others because you may not have much control over whether they happen. For example, you can't control aging forever, or prevent children from growing up and leaving home, or avoid having to move because of a job loss, or prevent experiencing a traumatic event. Still, you can try your best to reduce your chronic pain by choosing some of the following strategies that will help you cope better with life stressors.

1. Perceive each life stressor as a challenge or an opportunity to grow from confronting it and taking action, rather than catastrophizing (thinking nothing will change or that it's hopeless). Maintain your hope even if it takes weeks, perhaps months to change.

2. Prioritize all life stressors that are higher than a 7 on the Life Stress Pain Scale. Once you've prioritized them, then start with the most important ones to reduce, then work your way down the list.

3. Clarify whether each high-scaled life stressor is a crisis that may have a significant impact on your pain level in the immediate future. If it is, you need to work fast to deal with the stressor head-on, since time becomes a critical factor. If not, then you can still follow the strategies below, but focus less on the need for immediate change and more on strategic planning.

4. Use meditation and relaxation skills while trying to reduce life stressors. Intermittent breaks to relax, de-stress and regroup are important for refueling so you can deal with life stressors.

5. Think of how you and others you know have coped well with similar life stressors in the past. Which strategies worked well? Can you apply similar strategies to the stressors you face now?

6. What information do you need to obtain to help you figure out a clear plan to reduce these stressors? Having more knowledge about dealing with the life stressor can help you feel more in control of it. Gather as much information as you can to handle whatever comes your way.

7. Consider establishing sub-goals for specific time periods. For example, what can you accomplish today to help you reduce these life stressors? How about in a week? A month? Two months? Six months? A year?

8. Build your network of support. Who or what systems can you rely on to help you cope with life stressors?

9. Consider delegating responsibilities as a way of coping with the life stressors. You have nothing to lose by making requests. You'll find that most people are willing to help when they know you are confronting major stressors in your life.

10. What aspects of the life stressors can you control, and what aspects are beyond your control? It's easier to think of plans for the ones you can control. Develop and rehearse self-coaching statements to deal with those aspects of the life stressors you cannot control.

11. Focus on using your assertiveness skills. You have the rights to say "No," to make requests, to state your opinions, to express your feelings, to disagree, and to do only what you are humanly capable of doing.

12. Monitor how well you are doing on reducing life stressors by using the Life Stressor Scale on a weekly basis.

13. There will often be some life stressors that you cannot change but for which you can generate positive rationalizations, so as to accept that you may have no control over the situation.

14. Know the common symptoms most people experience when confronting a traumatic event. These include physical, thinking, and emotional symptoms.

15. Becoming upset about a life stressor will increase your pain. Try to do whatever it takes to get your stress levels down to 1 to 4 by doing mindfulness exercises, using self-calming statements, tapping into visual imagery of peaceful scenes, or taking periodic breaks.

16. If you are experiencing a lot of tension between you and significant others about resolving a major life stressor, then I would suggest that you try to resolve your conflict by meeting in a controlled environment, like a food court or some other public place where there are many people around. You may feel more comfortable trying to think of ways to resolve your conflict without shouting or yelling at one another.

17. If you are experiencing much tension about a major life stressor, don't involve your children or teenagers in your discussions with your significant other. They will experience further stress if they hear you having intense arguments. While they need to appreciate that conflicts over life stressors can be resolved in healthy ways, they don't need to get involved in them.

18. Do not try to get other people who are not involved in your conflict to agree with you. It is not fair to try to have uninvolved parties take sides.

19. If you still cannot resolve your conflict over major life stressors, then get help from a therapist or a mediator who specializes in couples therapy or conflict resolution.

20. Remember that just because you are unable to change a particular life stressor, it doesn't mean you are always helpless or a helpless person.

21. You may not be the pilot of your plane, but you can trust that the pilot will get you through the turbulence. What you can do is take control of the dials on the instrument panel (the five scales) that help strengthen the plane's capacity to navigate through the storm.

In the next chapter, we'll focus on ways to reduce the emotional component of chronic pain.

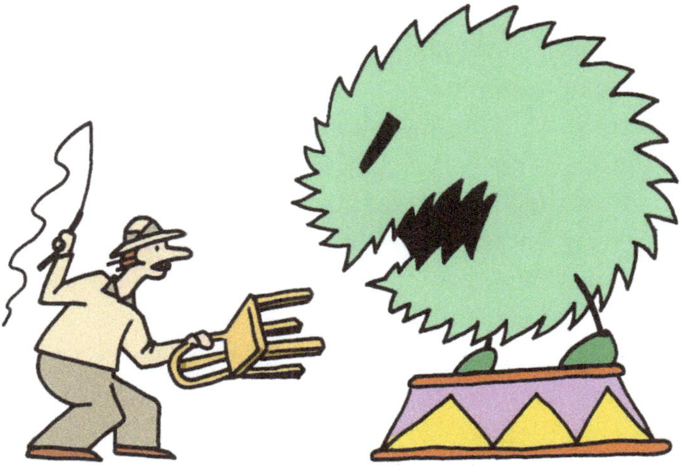

Fight back no matter how tough it looks.

Chapter 9: Ways to Reduce Your Emotional Pain

Beyond physical causes and life stressors, pain can also have an emotional component. There are different categories of emotional pain, and this chapter provides suggestions for handling and reducing these. All the strategies identified in this chapter are based on my professional and personal experiences. Choose the ones that you feel may work best for you.

Fight Depression

Nearly everyone experiences different levels of depression and other emotions, even on a day-to-day basis. Just because you feel very depressed (a rating between 7 and 10) today doesn't mean you'll feel that way every day. So, be careful of all-or-nothing thinking that you express as, "I'm always depressed." Rather, focus on all the days you weren't depressed but simply felt sad or disappointed or, more importantly, focus on the days when you feel happy and optimistic.

If, however, you are rating your feelings of depression between a seven and a ten, almost on a daily basis, your emotional pain level is severe and it implies that you are very depressed and in need of immediate help. You are probably feeling hopeless and helpless. You need to talk to a mental health professional immediately if you are having any thoughts or specific plans of harming yourself or someone else. Have a person close to you drive you to the nearest hospital emergency room. You will be evaluated by an on-call clinician to determine if you aren't safe enough and need to be admitted to a psychiatric inpatient unit. Most units are typically short-term with a team that does a diagnostic evaluation, manages medication, facilitates goal-setting and coping skills groups. This is typically followed on discharge by a partial day treatment program, then intensive outpatient therapy.

Consider getting on a medication that helps with depression if your ratings are consistently higher than seven. This may be a selective serotonin reuptake inhibitor (SSRI) like fluoxetine (Prozac), sertraline (Zoloft), citalopram (Celexa) or escitalopram (Lexapro); a selective serotonin norepinephrine reuptake inhibitor (SSNRI) like duloxetine (Cymbalta) or venlafaxine HCL (Effexor); or a medicine like bupropion (Wellbutrin) or a tricyclic antidepressant (TCA) like amitriptyline HCL (Elavil). Some of these medicines can also help with pain and anxiety. Mood stabilizers like Lithobid (lithium carbonate) or valproic acid (Depakoate) may be prescribed for more severe, mood disorder conditions like bipolar disorder. Often, new antipsychotics or anti-seizure medications can have a positive effect on mood stability. In this category are medications like lamitrogine (Lamictal), aripiprazole (Abilify) or quetiapine (Seroquel). Other medications like Neurontin or Lyrica can help ease neuropathic pain.

Look at your daily activity schedule for the week. If you find that you have many unscheduled activities or have planned activities that give you little in the way of feeling mastery and/or pleasure, chances are that this is contributing greatly to your high ratings of depression. Consequently, plan more masterful or pleasurable activities into your schedule.

Pay close attention to specific life stressors that are getting you down. Do whatever it takes to lower them by implementing adaptive coping strategies, like implementing S.M.A.R.T. goals with time frames, using positive self-talk, and establishing better support systems.

Be aware if you are self-medicating (i.e., using various substances to dull physical, cognitive or emotional pain), and instead try to ease your difficulty with fortitude skills. It is very common to have a dual or even triple diagnosis of pain, mood disorders, and substance abuse, so be aware if this is occurring.

Make sure the professional on your pain management team is licensed and trained in pain management, mood disorders, and substance abuse disorders.

Focus on your negative thoughts, then transform them into rational thoughts to reduce depressive feelings. Review the common negative cognitive thoughts that increase depressive conditions in Chapter 10 and use the recommended thought record similar to the one created by Aaron Beck to write down rational thoughts to improve your mood.

Use thought stopping and distraction to counter negative thoughts that fuel depression. Simply say to yourself, "Stop it!" or have a symbol like a red dot or stop sign help you to remember.

Think of all the ways your situation could be worse (unless you think like this too much, as that could mean you are more anxious than relieved).

Control Anxiety

Rating a moderate level of anxiety (ratings of 4 to 6) is a healthy range for you. Having some level of anxiety can help you to initiate action when solving problems or making healthy choices. Too little anxiety (ratings of 1 to 3) can mean that you may be unaware of situations that could be unhealthy or dangerous and on which you need to take some kind of action. Having too little anxiety can lead you to act before thinking about the consequences of your actions. The opposite situation can also be a problem. Having too much ongoing anxiety can mean you are experiencing some form of anxiety disorder. High levels of anxiety can increase your muscle tension, blood pressure or deregulate your sugar or cortisol levels.

Find out whether there is a genetic predisposition to anxiety disorders in your extended family. Do you or your relatives suffer from some forms of generalized anxiety, including constant futuristic, catastrophic worry or possible symptoms like restlessness, sweatiness, light-headedness, or a choking sensation? It's possible to have panic attacks that last anywhere from a few minutes to hours and come on randomly. There's also agoraphobia, a fear of open places and a tendency to avoid leaving "secure" places like home. Obsessive-compulsive symptoms include thoughts or urges that you know are silly but believe you must think or act on repetitively. If this sounds like your situation, you may need to be on a medication that has been shown to be helpful for long-term anxiety.

Like depressive symptoms, anxiety symptoms can be masked by the use of substances like alcohol or drugs. People often self-medicate, especially since pain management teams are cutting back on the distribution of benzodiazepines like diazepam (Valium) and lorazepam (Ativan) because of the potential for patients to become dependent on them. Be open with your pain management team about recognizing whether or not this is true for you.

Learn how to relax. Use breathing techniques practiced in yoga or when doing tai chi or listen to relaxation strategies shared on certain applications, podcasts or CDs where you learn how to focus on reducing muscle tension in your body. One such practice is the body scan: you learn to relax each muscle in your body, starting from your feet, through your legs, hips, chest and arms until you reach your head. Another way is to simply notice any area of your body where you feel tension, then try to focus on relaxing that particular area. Practice doing this in a quiet place for at least 10 minutes.

Another relaxation strategy is to simply find or imagine a relaxing, peaceful scene or simply focus on a monotone sound (like the hum of a fan) or watch a candle glow. Try to avoid thinking or judging. Simply use your senses to become aware of your surroundings.

Practice the mindfulness meditation strategies recommended in Chapter 11.

Distraction is a critical component in reducing anxiety. Do something to take your mind away from troubling or negative thoughts and physical symptoms by focusing on something outside of yourself. Practice a hobby like playing a musical instrument, enjoy a game of cards or do a crossword puzzle. You can also color, crochet or bird-watch. Take an interest in others instead of over-focusing on your pain.

The strategy of thought-stopping (catching yourself having anxious thoughts) is a useful technique to help you reduce them. Use a counting device to count the number of times you have an anxious thought within a certain time period. Then try to reduce that number over time, but make sure you set realistic, incremental sub-goals.

Review the common negative thinking errors described in the next chapter that increase anxiety states. Use the strategies identified to first catch yourself engaging in these thinking errors, then generate rational responses that will help you to reduce anxiety.

Cool Anger

Becoming and remaining angry is counterproductive to reducing your pain. If anything, remaining angry can increase your pain and can push others away. Your anger can be a defense against your acknowledging other, more vulnerable feelings such as feeling hurt, pained, vulnerable or misunderstood.

Try to use these next few suggestions to help reduce your anger ratings over time.

Cool down! If you feel like you're getting too hot and will react emotionally, then it's clear you've got to cool down quickly before you say or do things you'll regret later.

How does your body signal that you are feeling like you are ready to say or do something that you may regret? Know your physical signals that especially increase your desire to shout, scream, yell, hit, or throw something.

Try any of the following to cool down:

- Deep breathing, focusing on each inhale and exhale and counting slowly from 1 to 10, saying the next consecutive number with each exhale.
- Say in your head, "Cool down," "Chill," or "Stay calm."
- Take a break! Get away from the scene to calm down and give yourself a chance to think more clearly.

Be careful that your response of becoming angry is not a result of "mind reading" or projecting your thoughts and feelings onto someone else. This can be a result of having low self-esteem and thinking, "That person thinks I don't know anything," when it may really mean, "I don't think I know anything."

If someone becomes angry at you, try to respond this way: "What is it about ___ that's making you get so angry?" or "What are other reasons why ___ is becoming angry at me (i.e., hurt, pained, misunderstood)?"

Often, anger can result from a misperception, a miscommunication or a distortion. Reflect on whether any of these conditions may be contributing to your feeling angry.

Recognize the medical hazards of becoming angry. It's no different than slamming on your accelerator pedal while your car is in neutral. Anger will quickly increase the reactions from the sympathetic nervous system. These include an increase in blood pressure and heart rate, rapid breathing, muscle constriction, and/or an increase in adrenalin and cortisol.

Feelings of anger are often a defense against underlying feelings of pain, helplessness, a loss of control, or vulnerability. Try to recognize what you're truly feeling instead of simply getting angry.

If your feelings of anger are related to a lack of healthy assertiveness, then use the strategies identified in Chapter 11 for improving assertiveness on the Fortitude Scale.

Realize that becoming angry can push others away. Try to use statements like, "I feel hurt when...." or "I am pained when..." These are more vulnerable feelings to share with someone else, but you'll notice others are more willing to listen and respond to what you're thinking and feeling.

Increase Happiness

Most people learn how to be happy. Martin Seligman, a psychologist and researcher, identified major ways to improve one's happiness after studying how animals experience "learned helplessness" and become depressed by having no way to avoid pain. Seligman changed his perspective radically to focus on how to improve happiness. Review the following strategies to increase your happiness.

I suggest you read the book *Authentic Happiness* by Martin Seligman, the founder of the field of "positive psychology." In his book, Seligman identifies the virtues of happiness and how to obtain and enhance them.

Visit Dr. Seligman's website, www.authentichappiness.org, where you can do assessments to identify your signature strengths and read about how to develop a positive perspective about your chronic pain.

Try smiling as much as you can during the day. Notice how much just the act of smiling connects you to others and makes you feel better.

Listen to songs that have lyrics that make you feel happy and inspired, or to music that makes you feel good. Every morning, I listen to music composed by J.S. Bach. Find your favorite composers and listen to their music. Make a playlist of songs that refer to happiness. Some examples include:

"Don't Worry! Be Happy!"
"Put on a Happy Face"
"Tomorrow"
"The Impossible Dream"
"Climb Every Mountain"
"Singing in the Rain"

Be happy about the simple things in life. Just the fact that you are able to get up, breathe, and use your senses should be enough to make you happy. Be happy even when you accomplish small goals in your pain reduction strategy.

Do something kind for someone else at least once weekly. The more you perform acts of kindness for others, the more you will experience happiness and meaningfulness.

Happiness, optimism and gratitude are interrelated. See Chapter 11 for ways to increase optimism and gratitude.

You can increase your happiness by simply changing the way you think. In the next chapter, you'll discover ways to further reduce your pain by reducing your negative thinking.

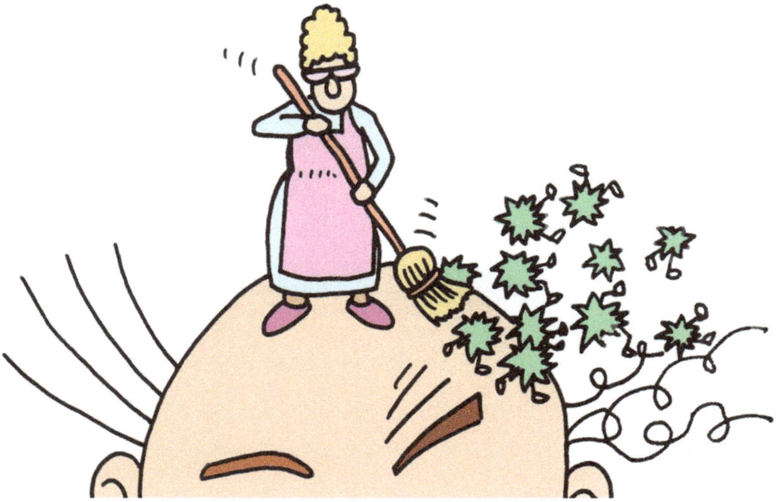

Sweep away those bad thoughts.

Chapter 10: Ways to Reduce Your Pain from Negative Thinking

Research by Aaron Beck and his colleagues has confirmed that that there is a strong relationship between how you think and how you feel. If you can change your negative thinking, you will change your negative emotional states. This applies to thoughts about your chronic pain.

Utilize the automatic thought record on pages 124-125 to keep a journal of ways to change your negative thinking. In turn, you will see a positive change in your pain levels.

First, note the date and time of your experience in columns one and two. Next, describe the situation in column three. In column four, identify your automatic thoughts and their relationship to how strongly you are feeling something on a scale of 0-100, with 0 meaning you have no feeling and 100 meaning you feel this strongly. After writing down your automatic thought(s) on the situation, identify in column five what common negative thoughts listed below are associated with your written thought(s). Use the relevant questions associated with the common negative thoughts below to write down a rational response to the same situation in column six. Note how much you believe your rational responses to be true. Finally, re-rate your feeling state, using the same scale of 0-100. What difference do you notice in your pain level if you have a rational response to the same situation?

AUTOMATIC THOUGHT RECORD

Date/ Time	Describe Stressful Situation	Emotional/ Physical change 0-100%	Automatic negative thought(s) (How much do you believe it (them) to be true? 0-100%

What is the cognitive appraisal to each negative, automatic thought?	Rational response(s) - Use adapative questions to compose alternative rational response(s) to the stressful situation.	1. How much do you believe the rational response(s) to be true? 0-100% 2. Emotional/Physical change 0-100?

Adapted by the author from materials by Aaron Beck, MD

Let's turn now to a dozen different ways to reduce your pain from having negative thoughts.

1. All-or-Nothing (Dichotomous) Thinking: Ask yourself these questions: Am I thinking in all-or-nothing ways? Do I see that there is a grey area? How realistic is it to think this way based on the evidence? How probable is it that things will turn out the way I am thinking?

2. Overgeneralization: How realistic is my conclusion? Is it based on objectivity? Evidence? Have there been times in the past when positive experiences occurred that were the opposite of my conclusion? Are there activities I still can do that go against my conclusion? How is it that my overall self-worth is measured by one mistake or by not meeting one goal?

3. Mental Filtering: Am I filtering in only negative information that fits my assumption? How objective, reliable or valid is this? Are there other possible positive conclusions I can come to instead of a negative one? Does one bad apple really spoil the whole bunch?

4. Disqualifying the Positive: Why emphasize the negatives? What have been my achievements, however small, rather than my limitations? Is it possible to lower my self-standards? After all, I am human!

5. Futuristic Thinking (Jumping to conclusions): How probable is it that what I am concerned about will occur? What does the history of similar situations tell me? Is it just as likely to be a positive outcome? So what if it turns out negative? Then what? How much control do I really have over determining how it will be? Is it possible to simply not know? To what extent does thinking about the future take me away from appreciating each moment in time? Can I be mindful of each moment, using my senses without judgment?

6. Catastrophizing (Magnification): How probable is it that my imagined catastrophe is likely to happen? Is there an equally probable positive outcome? What do my past experiences show? How much control do I really have to determine the future? What are the consequences of thinking of the worst-case scenario?

7. Emotional Reasoning: Am I being rational, logical, objective, realistic? Have there been times when I felt something was true and it turned out to be incorrect?

8. "Should" Statements: Is this thought based on a realistic, rather than an idealistic self-standard? Is it possible to lower my self-standards to some degree? Do I have a healthy balance between "shoulds" and "loves" or "desires"? Is the "should" based on my affirming that I'm doing "enough"? In what ways do "should" statements impact my self-esteem?

9. Labeling: What is the evidence to conclude that I should judge myself in such a harsh manner? Why am I my own worst enemy? Do others perceive me to be this way?

10. Need for Control: How much control do I really have over everything in life? Are there alternative, realistic reasons why I don't have control over this situation? How human is it to feel helpless at times? Just because I feel helpless now, does it mean I'll always feel helpless (all-or-nothing thinking) or that I'm inadequate (Labeling)?

11. Personalization: How much responsibility do I really have for something? What are alternative explanations that have nothing to do with me? What is the evidence to prove otherwise? What is the rationale for being so hard on myself?

12. Underestimating Strengths: Why am I focusing only on my vulnerabilities and not on my strengths? What skills or abilities did I possess before that allowed me to have coped well in similar situations?

You've now had an opportunity to see how, by improving your thinking, you can change how you feel and, in turn, decrease your pain. At this point, we will turn to the last section of the book, which focuses on improving your fortitude, or your courage to handle pain.

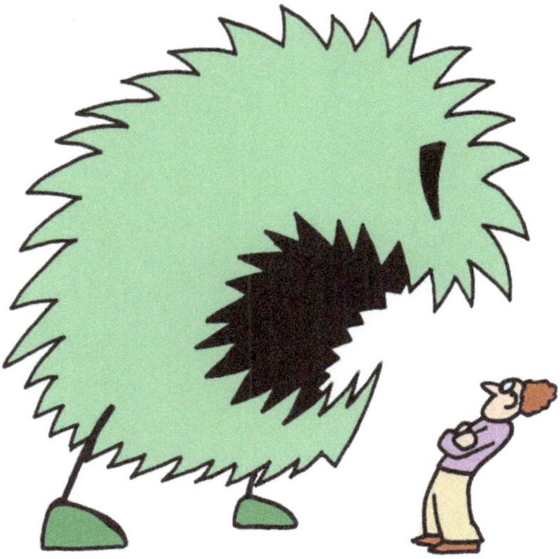

Be more like David, and defeat Goliath.

Chapter 11: Ways to Reduce Pain by Improving Fortitude Skills

"Patience and fortitude conquer all things."
-Ralph Waldo Emerson

"Out of suffering comes the serious mind;
Out of salvation the grateful heart;
Out of endurance, fortitude;
Out of deliverance, faith;
Patient endurance attends to all things."
-Teresa of Avila

You will reduce pain by increasing your ability to endure hardships. Your ability to perceive your pain as a challenge, rather than a hardship, will transform how you handle it. Once you improve your ratings on the sixteen fortitude skills covered in this chapter, you will realize that your pain can be overcome, and that you can decrease adversity.

Explore each of the seventeen skills and then determine which strategies you will use to transform the ways you handle pain into pursuing a positive Pain Management Lifestyle.

Seventeen Skills for Your Fortitude Tool Kit	
Coping Skills	Cognitive Flexibility
Self-Care	Optimism
Self-Efficacy	Humor
Assertiveness	Resilience
Exercise	Gratitude
Distraction	Supportive Systems
Mindfulness	Love
Problem-Solving	Spirituality
Self-Monitoring	

Coping Skills

"In three words I can sum up everything I've learned about life. It goes on."
~ Robert Frost

Your ability to confront upsets and disappointments is a critical factor in reducing your chronic pain. It's become harder these days since the rapid advancements in technology have contributed to people wanting things immediately. Faster is not necessarily better. Improving your coping skills is simply the ability to refine the skills you've been using since you learned them in childhood. Choose from the following strategies the ones that work for you.

1. Reflect on adaptive ways you've dealt with frustrations and disappointments related to experiencing chronic pain in the past. Utilize the strategies you've learned from previous experiences. These should include adaptive thoughts, positive self-talk and actions.

2. Reflect on positive role models you've either encountered personally or heard or read about over time. Reflect on the adaptive ways these people coped well with upsetting situations, especially chronic pain. What skills or abilities did they have? What did they value that helped them earn your respect?

3. Write down and rehearse positive, inspirational quotes or song lyrics, or read stories that reflect positive virtues about how to handle upsets, especially when it concerns coping with pain.

4. Each morning, create your day by thinking about, then writing down, how you're going to be. For example, you can write down "Be positive all day" or "Cope well with my pain" or "Be patient with ___." You'll be surprised how creating your day this way, starting your statement with the word "be," will help you remain consistent.

5. Try to smile all day. Smile and say hello to as many of the people as you meet that you can.

6. Prepare in advance for potential cognitive, emotional or physical triggers that can induce you to not cope well. Develop and keep strategic plans in place should you encounter such triggers.

7. Rehearse how you're going to cope adaptively to these triggers. Write down a sufficient number of "if-then" scenarios you may encounter.

8. Don't react! First calm down! Take a time-out, a quick break or even retreat if you can. Then, think the situation through before you decide on a way to cope. Use diaphragmatic (deep) breathing or do a mindfulness exercise first.

9. Use your support network. This could be anyone you can call, text or email, especially if you're feeling vulnerable to not coping well with your pain.

10. Be your own best coach when it comes to coping with chronic pain.

11. Use higher-level coping strategies like sublimation and humor. Write in a journal or create poems, short stories, song lyrics, fiction or non-fiction books. Draw, paint, sing, play an instrument, listen to music. Attend concerts and plays; watch comedies, old and new. Read or listen to books, especially biographies of those who've endured pain.

12. Remember that your situation could be a lot worse compared to situations others are facing, for example.

13. Rehearse and use daily positive self-coping statements like the following:
    - "Be brave and carry on despite the pain."
    - "I can overcome the pain."
    - "I won't let my pain stand in the way of what I want to do."
    - "I can handle this."
    - "Stay relaxed."
    - "Live one moment at a time."
    - "Never give up."

14. Rehearse and use daily words of inspiration like the following:
    - "Success is the sum of small efforts, repeated day in and day out." Robert Collier
    - "To climb steep hills requires a slow pace at first." Shakespeare
    - "While there is life, there is hope." Cicero
    - "You can because you think you can." Virgil
    - "Hope is a waking dream." Aristotle
    - "Never lose hope." Unknown
    - "Pain happens but suffering is optional." Unknown

Self-Care

"Until you value yourself, you won't value your time. Until you value your time, you will not do anything with it."
M. Scott Peck

Self-care is a key component of self-esteem. Here are ways to improve your self-esteem and thus improve your fortitude skills.

1. Take a sheet of paper and divide it into two parts. On the left side, make a list of things you have to do. On the right side, list the things you'd love to do or have passion for doing. Now, focus on developing a commitment to the activities on the right side of your sheet that is just as strong as the left side. Try to balance the sheet as much as possible.

2. Don't let rationalizations become obstacles that keep you from doing things you'd love to do, so long as they're objectively realistic, timely and cost-effective.

3. Reaffirm your commitment with statements like, "I deserve to do ___" or "I work hard enough to enjoy ___."

4. Generate a support system to help yourself begin and continue self-care activities.

5. Be wary of all-or-nothing thinking or labeling. Just because you care for yourself doesn't mean you're "selfish" or never care for others. Even cars need refueling to keep going, and people are no different.

6. If you're not used to initiating self-care activities, then get your feet wet a little at a time. Try doing certain activities for short time periods or try activities that wouldn't make you feel too guilty about taking time for yourself. Then begin to increase these activities over time so that you find a healthy balance between self-care activities and those that give you sense of mastery or self-efficacy.

7. If you tend to be a perfectionist, then transform the use of the word "should." Try saying things to yourself like, "I should relax!" or "I should care for myself!" or "I should reward myself by doing something nice for myself after doing some must-do task!"

Self-Efficacy

Self-efficacy is the extent to which you derive satisfaction from accomplishing things. These things could range from completing small projects around the house to writing a poem to making regular donations of time or needed items at a local food pantry or animal shelter.

1. Know your skills or abilities. (every one of us has many) rather than telling yourself that you have none. Review a list of common skills or abilities, then rate yourself on each skill from 1 to 5, with 5 meaning you definitely have this skill and 1 meaning you definitely don't have this skill. A good starter list of skills can be found in *What Color Is Your Parachute?* (2017) by Richard Bolles.

2. Do those activities that give you a sense of accomplishment and satisfaction. Rate those activities on a scale of 1-5 (with 1 indicating little sense of accomplishment and 5 indicating a strong feeling of accomplishment), and then try to do activities that you have rated as higher than a 3.

3. Make sure the activities you identify are realistic and definable. If not, then break down activity goals into sub-goals.

4. Be proud of your accomplishments. Reward yourself with a self-care activity after completing each self-efficacy activity, even if it's a sub-goal.

5. Learn about your pain. Knowledge helps you to be more in control of your pain. There is always more to learn, but don't become stuck with the cognitive error of "I don't know enough." That will only make you feel inadequate and anxious, especially if you're a perfectionist. Instead, learn as much as you can while realizing learning is an ongoing process through life. Focus on what you do know instead of on what you don't know.

6. The more you do things for satisfaction and accomplishment, the higher will be your level of confidence and rating on your resilience on the Fortitude Scale.

Assertiveness

"Too many of us fail to fulfill our needs because we say no rather than yes, yes when we should say no."
– William Glasser

Assertiveness is another way to increase fortitude. Your ability to say what you think, to change your mind and, to say, "No!" will help you build confidence and lower your pain.

Recognize that your rights include the following; credit for items 1 through 10 goes to Manuel J. Smith.

1. The right to judge your own behavior, thoughts, and emotions, and to take the responsibility for their initiation and consequences upon yourself.
2. The right to offer no reasons or excuses for justifying your behavior.
3. The right to judge if you are responsible for finding solutions to other people's problems.
4. The right to change your mind.
5. The right to make mistakes—and be responsible for them.
6. The right to say, "I don't know."
7. The right to be independent of the goodwill of others before coping with them.
8. The right to be illogical in making decisions.
9. The right to say, "I don't understand."
10. The right to say, "I don't care."
11. The right to state what you think.
12. The right to state how you feel.
13. The right to disagree
14. The right to make requests.
15. The right to not tolerate any kind of abuse.
16. The right to care for yourself.
17. The right to be treated with respect
18. The right to feel good about yourself.
19. The right to be in trusting relationships.
20. The right to feel good.

Keep an assertiveness journal. Identify the date and time of the situation, including who or what was involved and what you heard, saw or read, which of the above rights was being violated, how you responded, and what the consequence was.

Assert yourself using the DESC acronym, which stands for Describe, Emote, Specify, Consequence.

1. Describe: Write down or say what you saw, heard or read as if you are a newspaper reporter simply noting the facts. For example, "John, this is the fifth time today that you told me to forget about the pain."

2. Emote: Express how what you saw, heard or read made you feel. For example, "I feel hurt that you don't seem to appreciate the level of pain I am in."

3. Specify a request. For example, "I'm asking that you stop saying that and be more understanding of what I am going through."

4. Consequence: Make an "if-then" statement. For example, "If you stop saying that and support me in an understanding way, then I'll feel closer to you."

Rehearse potential situations you believe may occur using assertiveness steps described by the DESC acronym. If you feel overwhelmed by feelings in a situation, take a time-out to calm down by doing some deep breathing or some mindfulness exercise. Practice the DESC script, and then return to the situation to assert yourself.

Take additional time to calm down to think through what you want to say or write.

Try not to "take the bait" if you believe your rights are being violated and you believe you are being set up to respond inappropriately or are about to respond ineffectively to a high-stress statement or action by another. Use time-outs to think things through when you need them. Think before you respond and re-check what you want to say or write. Get a reality check on how you're going to respond by getting feedback from other people. This is especially true with instant messaging, texting, or commenting on social media platforms. Try to use cool-down comments or humor to manage any heightened tension.

Exercise

"We are what we repeatedly do. Excellence then is not an act but a habit."
-- Aristotle

There is nothing better than exercise to get a natural high from the release of your bodies' natural endorphins. If you can swim or ride a stationary bike for thirty-five minutes, then do it! Be careful of all the reasons that can get in the way of exercising. Consider these strategies to increase your fortitude:

Don't give up, no matter what, even if you can do just a little physical activity every day or every few days.

Collaborate with your pain management team to design a realistic exercise program based on your pain levels and what you can tolerate. Please get a careful assessment done before beginning any type of exercise. Focus on improving your endurance, stability, mobility, and strength.

Stretch after you exercise. Again, review with your team to identify the best stretches based on your condition.

Try to set up a daily routine that may include walking where you can sit to take frequent breaks as needed

Develop a support team. Consider exercising with at least one other person. It's great when you can coach each other to exercise. Walking or doing other exercise with a friend makes it seem less strenuous.

Distraction

"All profound distraction opens certain doors."
-- Julio Cortazar

Taking time to simply get away from it all is a healthy way to reduce pain. Even the best sports coach knows when to call a time-out to have the team regroup to gain perspective and re-focus. Here are some strategies that you may find helpful.

Focus on activities that distract you from becoming preoccupied by negative thoughts, worrying, or withdrawing excessively. These activities could be anything: hobbies, reading, listening to talk shows, playing an instrument, taking an interest in someone else, doing good deeds, playing a game or doing a crossword puzzle, watching a movie or a sports event, or taking a course or webinar.

Structure your days so that you can gain both mastery and pleasure from these activities that distract you from your chronic pain.

Use a mindfulness exercise as described below in the next section of this chapter.

Mindfulness

"The present moment is filled with joy and happiness.
If you are attentive, you will see it."
-- Thich Nhat Hanh

The term "mindfulness meditation" has been around for centuries. The methodology has simply been reframed, perhaps for marketing purposes. Buddhist monks have practiced the steps over time, like focusing on the present, being still within a peaceful environment, and concentrating on one's breath. Other religious groups have done so as well.

Review the strategies below and choose the ones that fit the best for you.

If you enjoy reading, I would strongly recommend *The Relaxation Response* by Herbert Bensen (1975). I find this to be the best book to help you learn the key ingredients and benefits for any type of meditational exercise. Several other books to consider reading are, *Peace is Every Step* by Thich Nhat Hanh (1990), and *Mindfulness for Beginners* (2006) and *Full Catastrophe Living* (1990) by Jon Kabat-Zinn. The latter book is especially helpful because it is based on Zinn's work at the Stress Reduction Program at the University of Massachusetts Medical Center. If you really want to go back in time to experience the origins of modern-day mindfulness meditation practice, please read, *Zen Mind, Beginner's Mind* (1970) by Suzuki and *Be Here Now* (1978) by Baba Ram Dass (Richard Alpert).

Here are the keys to mindfulness meditation:

- Focus on your present sensory awareness -- just using your senses: what you see, hear, smell, taste and touch, moment by moment.
- Diaphragmatic (deep) breathing or visualization: Simply sit in a chair or lie down in a quiet area. Then close your eyes and breathe in, and breathe out, as deeply as you can, saying to yourself "in" or "one" on the in-breath and "out" or "two" on the out-breath. If you prefer visualization, imagine the ocean receding from the shoreline or rich blue-colored air when you

inhale, and the waves breaking on the shore or grey-colored air when you exhale.

- Avoidance of judgment: Stop any kind of thinking, especially judgments. If you find your mind wandering, then try to stop it and bring yourself back to focusing on your diaphragmatic breathing.

There are other ways to practice sensory awareness training as a means of meditation to reduce stress and chronic pain. For example, take pictures spontaneously with your phone camera. Find a scene or an object that appeals to you, then walk around snapping pictures that capture your vision. Again, focus on what you see without any judgment! Another practice is to take a sketchbook and draw something that you observe, perhaps a scenic area. Focus on your drawing and enjoy the motion of your hand and the feel of the paper and pencil. Try walking in a garden or greenhouse or near the ocean. Focus on your sense of smell. Hiking -- even short distances where you can stop at different points to rest -- is a great way to become fully aware of all your senses.

There are multiple applications and podcasts to help with learning and using meditation to calm the mind. Simply find the ones that work best for you.

Practice mindfulness meditation at least twice daily for a minimum of 10 minutes each session. Try this: first, rate your level of physical pain from 1-10, practice a mindfulness exercise, then re-rate your level of pain to see how much your pain level has decreased.

Problem-Solving Skills

"A sum can be put right: but only by going back
till you find the error and working it afresh from that point,
never by simply going on."
-- C.S. Lewis

Your ability to problem-solve is a gift that elevates you above all the other animals on this earth. It indicates how you are capable of reasoning and using your memory effectively to analyze a problem and resolve it, using the best steps you can think of, to form a conclusion. Choose from among these strategies to improve your rating on this element of the Fortitude Scale.

Identity the major problem you are facing, making sure it is not hiding a more important problem. Then think of all the ways you can deal with the problem, even if you must be patient with the fact that the problem cannot be solved right away. Then, weigh the pros and cons of each plan. You can do a cost-benefit analysis of each plan to solve the problem. You can do a cost-benefit analysis including a weighted score from 1-5 for each benefit and cost. Think of the benefits and costs of using specific plans, both short- and long-term. Then choose the best plan and act on it and evaluate how you did!

Prioritize your problems! Place the problems that relate to reducing your chronic pain into four categories:

1) Problems that need to be handled immediately or within the next 24 hours.
2) Problems that you can address within a week or two.
3) Problems that can be put off for a longer period of time.
4) Those problems you can delegate to others.

As you're thinking about how to solve your current problem, think of all the positive ways you've successfully handled past problems and reduced chronic pain. These can range from easy problems to moderately hard to difficult ones. They can be work-related problems, or family or interpersonal problems. What skills did it take for you to solve these problems well?

After you define the problem clearly, then identify what information you may need to obtain to help you define some ways to solve the problem. The more information you have, the more control you will have to eventually choose the best plan to reduce your pain.

Sometimes, the biggest problem can be that you aren't really clear on what the problem is. For example, the problem may be a function of a misperception, a misunderstanding, or a miscommunication. For example, you may think that the problem is that your husband doesn't care about your pain; that he's fed up with your acting as if you can't cope. What may be more accurate is that your husband is scared that you're acting as if you're giving up and that you don't want to live. In fact, he loves you and he doesn't want to lose you.

Use visualization techniques to problem-solve effectively. Close your eyes and imagine yourself reaching a positive solution to your problem. Now visualize going through all the steps to reach that solution. What steps did you envision going through to reach that positive outcome?

Emphasize what you did well when problem-solving. Be a supportive, encouraging self-coach, no matter how well you did. The worst-case scenario is that at least you tried!

It is the action that will bring you satisfaction or pleasure. Just do it! Don't get stuck in any one step in the sequence of problem-solving actions.

The better you are at problem-solving, the higher your resilience on the Fortitude Scale will be -- and that's important for your Pain Management Lifestyle.

Self-Monitoring

"Self-discipline is often disguised as short-term pain, which often leads to long-term gains. The mistake many of us make is the need and want for short-term gains (immediate gratification), which often leads to long-term pain."
-- Charles F. Glass

Think before you act! How easy it is to say this when we are being inundated with all kinds of ways to get something done right this second. Even buying items online takes just a push of a phone button rather than a drive to the shopping mall. The number of people becoming phone-addicted is rising dramatically. t's a blessing to slow down and weigh your options. It will reduce your pain, as well. Choose from the following strategies the ones that will work the best for you.

Having an "observing self" is key to reducing your chronic pain. From infancy, all of us have developed this inner capacity to talk to ourselves about situations and inner sensations. You learned this from developing the use of your memory and then the use of language to self-monitor your thoughts, feelings and actions. Listen to your "inner voice" and clarify whether it is helping to guide you to think and reason in adaptive ways. If your inner voice is not helpful in this way, then re-focus on how to reduce your negative thinking as measured on the Negative Cognitive Appraisal Scale.

Use all five of the pain rating scales at least once weekly to evaluate how you are doing to reduce chronic pain. Identify what has helped and what hasn't helped to change your ratings in a positive way.

Slow down when you're problem-solving or when managing your feelings. You must "stop and think" to give yourself more time to reduce your stress in the most effective possible way.

Listen to that "inner voice" that helps you to reflect first on the consequences before putting specific pain-reducing plans into action. To slow down and think it through is to regulate your impulses and see situations from a positive perspective.

Emphasize the last segment of problem-solving, asking yourself "How did I do?" to evaluate what you put into action to reduce chronic pain. Did it work or not?

Don't think too much or obsess. Excessive thinking will just make you more worried and anxious. You want to be confident in your evaluation, not preoccupied with doubt and self-criticism. This is especially true if you're a perfectionist who has high self-standards. Be a positive coach to yourself, not a constant critic!

Cognitive Flexibility

"The measure of intelligence is the ability to change."
-- Albert Einstein

You are often required to shift from one task to another. You may have difficulty with this task, especially if you are concentrating deeply on one, then are interrupted to change your focus on having to do something else. This can be quite difficult if you really like what you are doing and do not expect this sudden change. To reduce feelings of frustration and pain and to prevent possible arguments with significant people in your life who may ask you to "stop what you are doing and please help me with ___," I recommend that you consider choosing from the following strategies the ones that may best help you to increase your fortitude in this area.

One major executive function of the brain's prefrontal cortex is cognitive flexibility or cognitive shifting. This means that you have the ability to change course when meeting upsets or disappointments. You can be cognitively flexible, self-monitor your situation, then problem-solve and renew your coping ability.

Rather than become stuck in grieving your loss, accept your pain as a challenge. Regain your hope that all is not lost. Act in ways to reduce your pain so that the pain doesn't consume you. Then maintain your commitment to the specific pain management strategies you've chosen that prevent relapse. Build your capabilities to cope and reduce your chronic pain. You can always create new sub-goals rather than try to meet overly idealistic ones. If you lose five pounds, then setting another sub-goal of losing five more pounds can be attainable. If you are capable of walking a few blocks, then a revised goal can be walking a half-mile next time. Loving each moment can be amended to loving life.

Realize that you may have periodic upsets that impede your ability to reduce chronic pain. Having cognitive flexibility means that you can think about and implement ways to overcome any obstacles to reducing chronic pain.

Consider generating backup plans if things get in the way of the first plan you put into action.

Manage your anger when experiencing frustrations. Use calming techniques to stop and think before you react. Learn to be patient, yet assertive.

Be careful not to set unrealistically high standards, especially if you are perfectionistic. Try lowering your standards and being less hard on yourself.

Pay close attention to having high ratings of control on the Cognitive Appraisal of Pain Scale. Try to reframe not having control over situations as simply temporary experiences of helplessness as part of the human condition.

Read the Serenity Prayer often, even if you don't attend Alcoholics Anonymous (AA) or Narcotics Anonymous (NA) meetings. If you don't know it, here it is; you may address it to G-d or to any other power you choose: "Grant me the serenity to accept the things I cannot change; courage to change the things I can; and the wisdom to know the difference."

Optimism

"A pessimist sees the difficulty in every opportunity; the optimist sees every opportunity in every difficulty."
-- Winston Churchill

This quote from Winston Churchill best encapsulates the importance of cultivating optimism. Choose from among the following strategies the ones that may work for you to improve your optimism ratings on the Fortitude Scale.

In his book *Learned Optimism*, Martin Seligman writes about how optimism can be enhanced. Try to perceive your problems with chronic pain as being temporary, and view them as mostly controllable (or capable of being reduced). The third step is to understand that they are mostly specific to the situation rather than generalizable to all situations.

Optimistic people are happier than those people who think negatively and catastrophize about the future. Try to stop all negative thinking by using thought-stopping techniques. Pinch yourself or snap a rubber band around your wrist every time you have a negative thought, and say to yourself, "Stop it!" Or use visual cues like red dots or make a "stop sign" to remind yourself to stop and think.

To be optimistic is to have hope in a manner similar to hostages held in captivity for long periods of time. Do whatever it takes to instill hope, including reading or listening to anything inspirational.

Optimistic people let things go. Don't hold onto grudges or upsets with people. Apologize and work through as many conflicts as you can. Your experience of having chronic pain can make you more sensitive to what others say and do. Be careful that you don't mind-read, misunderstand or misperceive what is really going on between someone else and yourself.

Change the way you view obstacles to reducing chronic pain by seeing them as challenges or opportunities. Your challenges are a function of your life journey; think of them as a positive way to transform your negative thoughts, feelings, and actions.

Generate a positive probable outcome for every anticipated negative outcome of an action plan to reduce your chronic pain.

Try to smile as much as possible within yourself and towards others. You'll find that smiling is catchy and fuels positive connectedness with others.

Martin Seligman notes that instead of blaming themselves, optimists focus on the notion that factors beyond their control, due to circumstances or to someone else's actions, caused a negative experience. The more you can do this, the lower your rating should be on "control" on the Cognitive Appraisal of Pain Scale.

Humor

"A day without laughter is a day wasted."
-- Charlie Chaplin

In his book *Anatomy of an Illness as Perceived by the Patient*, Norman Cousins describes how ten minutes of laughter daily, as an adjunct to traditional treatment, helped him overcome what doctors believed was a one in a hundred chance of surviving an adrenal disease. Mr. Cousins believed that positive emotions could bring about well-being. In his life, Mr. Cousins used humor to avoid bypass surgery. Asked about these experiences, he said he believed humor was a powerful tool for reducing anxiety, panic, and helplessness.

Recognize the benefits of humor. It improves your immune system function, lowers your stress levels, and increases your positive outlook on life. Humor can increase your happiness and lower your ratings on depression, anxiety and anger on the Emotional Pain Scales. It can also increase your optimism and resilience on the Fortitude Scale.

As much as you can, avoid reading or listening to any news that increases your anger or despair. Instead, watch comedies, listen to funny talk shows, read and listen to jokes, funny stories, and satire. Laugh at the absurdities of life. Try to find jokes about coping with pain. As strange as this may sound, you may find the humor about pain to be a stress reliever.

Look for any opportunity to use humor in conversations. Everyone experiences some form of pain, whether it be due to physical causes, life stress, emotional states, negative cognitive appraisals or lack of fortitude. No one is exempt from pain. Use humor tactfully to help others reduce their life pain.

Be around people who have a good sense of humor. It brings you closer together.

Have the power to laugh at yourself rather than be self-critical. Disparagement theory is about the ability to laugh at ourselves and our human frailties.

Resilience

"Resilience is accepting your new reality, even if it's less good than the one you had before. You can fight it, you can do nothing but scream about what you've lost, or you can accept that and try to put together something that's good."
-- Elizabeth Edwards

Resilience is the ability to grow from painful experiences. The greater your resilience, the more effective you will be in overcoming setbacks and upsets.

Think of times when you were able to bounce back from having chronic pain. What abilities, virtues and strengths did you have that helped you bounce back? To what extent do you acknowledge yourself for having the ability to use these traits again to face future setbacks, should they occur?

Think of others you know who have had chronic pain and bounced back fairly well. What do you think it took for them to do so?

What happens when you have a setback? That's okay. Don't be too hard on yourself! It's no different than having a relapse. It may just be that some of your weekly monitored, negative scale ratings may increase or your positive ones may decrease. Remember that your overall goal of having a Pain Management Lifestyle is to improve your scale ratings over time. The essence is to try to focus on increasing the average number of healthy days or weeks between setbacks over time.

Recognize your triggers that induce setbacks. Often, they're related to increased negative thinking or feelings of anxiety, depression, or anger. Your triggers may be due to some life stressor beyond your control or it could simply be from an aggravated physical condition that may require you to seek a medical consult. When you have a setback, think about what you need to get back on track to improve your scale ratings.

Try to obtain support from caring others to help you re-group!

Make a list of times in your life when you confronted other challenges and were able to bounce back. These challenges could have been at any age, with family or friends, at school or work or when you were involved in different organizations. These challenges could have been about your health, a life stage crisis, or about your finances. After you list these challenges, think of what it took for you to bounce back.

As mentioned previously, a healthy sleep pattern is important to resilience. If you're not getting enough sleep, talk to your medical team about what may help you to sleep more effectively.

Think of ways you can increase meaningfulness in your life. How can you make a difference, gain satisfaction from helping others or help to promote an important cause?

Do what it takes to confront any fears or worries that may make you avoid taking steps to reduce your chronic pain. Review strategies to deal with negative thinking and excessive worry. If you have fears that relate to taking action to reduce chronic pain, then meet with a professional who can teach you muscle relaxation techniques that are associated with them. This process is called systematic desensitization.

Resilience and optimism are often correlated. That is, the more you maintain a positive outlook, the more resilient you may be. What are some positive words of encouragement you've said to yourself or heard others say that can help you improve your resilience and reduce your chronic pain ratings?

Make a list of your particular strengths and virtues. Review the list of major ones noted in the book *Authentic Happiness* (2002) by Martin Seligman.

Humor and resilience can often go together. To what extent can you use humor to deal with setbacks? Think of times in the past when you were able to get through difficult days using humor.

Do simple, enjoyable activities you've built into your day to help you improve your ability to bounce back from a situation and to help reduce your chronic pain.

Identify your support network of people you can rely on when you must overcome setbacks and improve your resilience.

Know which triggers tend to increase stress for you, whether it's anger or frustration. Note what you can do differently to lower your ratings on the anger and life stress scales and improve the ratings on the resilience scale.

Keep to some sort of daily routine to help reduce chronic pain.

Reframe your capacity to confront stress as a positive opportunity to grow from a challenge.

Gratitude

"Walk as if you are kissing the Earth with your feet."
-- Thich Nhat Hanh

Your being grateful goes a long way to offset the stresses, strains and worries that can consume your mind. To be grateful means to make your pain and suffering less of a focus than your happiness and pleasure. Be grateful even for the simplest things. Try it out! And you will see how being grateful each day reduces your chronic pain!

Get up each morning and express gratitude for the positive experiences you have in your life. Must you wait for Thanksgiving to express gratitude? It is easy for you to focus on your pain, your anger, your hurts, what you could have been or should have done rather than the things in your life that bring comfort, nurturance and meaningfulness?

It is imperative to get up each morning and express thanks for at least five things for which you are grateful. Make the list ongoing, even if you repeat certain things.

You can share how much you're grateful when praying, as in thanking G-d or a higher power for appreciating the gift of life, for giving you food for this earth, for giving you water to drink, and for giving you clothes to wear.

Gratitude goes a long way to offset the stresses, strains, and worries that can consume our minds.

To be grateful means to make pain and suffering less of a focus than happiness and pleasure... even for the simplest things.

Supportive Systems

"A best friend is the only one that walks into
your life when the world has walked out."
--Shannon L. Alder

You can have much difficulty living with pain alone. You can cry in agony in bed or, you can choose to have those you love understand and help you make better choices to reduce your pain. Having a healthy supportive system of family or coworkers or friends is no different than a person who is suffering from overeating or from abusing substances. Having people who care about your life challenge can be as fruitful as a blossoming spring tree.

Consider some of the following strategies to improve your supportive system.

Write down a list of people, groups or organizations that can help support you in your efforts to reduce chronic pain. This especially includes others who experience chronic pain and those caretakers who can empathize well with your situation.

You can gain support by reading or listening to positive, optimistic information by meeting directly with others or by phone, e-mail or by text, by joining online supportive networks or by attending workshops or joining a free support group in your area.

Obtain ongoing support from members of your medical team. This includes seeing a licensed therapist who specializes in pain management on a regular basis, even if it's for periodic check-ins.

If you cannot make a scheduled on-site therapy, then consider tele-health, whereby your insurance company will pay for you to receive help through an online, secure video program. If your insurance plan doesn't allow this, then I'd suggest you contact your insurance representative and advocate for their endorsing it.

Participate! Don't create reasons to avoid connecting with others, especially those who are quite knowledgeable about chronic pain. You are not alone in having chronic pain!

Love

"The capacity to care is the thing which gives life its deepest significance."
-- Pablo Casals

Love is a powerful force in reducing chronic pain. Start with considering "Emuna" which, in Hebrew means an unconditional belief and faith that everything emanates from G-d. To love G-d and to know G-d loves you because he created you is a primary way to experience Divine Love. In the Old Testament, it is written, "And you shall Love the Lord thy G-d, with all thy heart, with all thy soul and with all thy might." In the New Testament, love emanates from the sayings of Jesus and his disciples. In the Quran, love is derived from one's direct relationship with Allah, based on the writings of the Prophet Mohammad. Read the sayings of Buddha and Confucius as they apply to love.

If any of these sources are uncomfortable for you to believe in, then consider having faith in a higher power or spiritual forces like those revered by Native Americans, or natural forces that emanate around you and in the universe.

If you still can't connect to this belief, then simply skip this item.

Love thyself! Self-love is a healthy form of primary narcissism that develops in an infant's interactions with others who fuel love and trust. To love yourself means to care for yourself; self-love does not mean being selfish. Rather, it is a major source of fuel for establishing a balance between nurturing yourself and caring for others.

Reflect on what you wrote down for self-care on the Fortitude Scale. Use that list as a way of experiencing love for yourself.

Make a list of all the people you love and have loved in your lifetime. Next to the name of each person, write down what it is about that person that you love or have loved so much. Then ask, "How can I apply those admirable qualities to myself?"

Try to tell at least one person a day that you love them. If this is too much, then try to do so once a week.

Show compassion for others. Help others in need; especially those who are suffering from chronic pain. Share with them that they are not alone. Be kind and do good deeds. Avoid judging people as you don't judge yourself.

Listen to the lyrics of love songs or read poems, essays, and stories about love.

Seek forgiveness. To forgive others or oneself can be quite a challenge. This may come especially hard if you have been the victim of trauma, including experiencing or witnessing physical, sexual or emotional abuse and have chronic pain. In his book *Authentic Happiness*, Martin Seligman writes that there is a positive relationship between life satisfaction and your capacity to forgive. He cites a large Stanford University study which concluded that individuals who participated in a six-session, ninety-minute workshop on forgiveness experienced significantly less anger, less stress, greater optimism and better health than a randomly assigned control group.

Seeking forgiveness may come especially hard for those who have been the victims of abuse and have chronic pain. I would recommend that you read *Forgiveness: How to Make Peace with your Past and Get on with your Life* by Sidney and Susan Simon. Another book that may help you work through your pain, especially if you still feel angry or seek revenge, is *Forgiveness and Reconciliation: Theory and Application* by Everett L. Worthington Jr.

Spirituality

"Knock, And He'll open the door
Vanish, And He'll make you shine like the sun
Fall, And He'll raise you to the heavens
Become nothing, And He'll turn you into everything."
-Jalaluddin Rumi

Faith in G-d had been an ardent healer for many with chronic pain who attended some form of worship well into the 1950s and early 1960s. The inspirational leadership of President Franklin D. Roosevelt from the Great Depression through World War II, and then John F. Kennedy, both of whom suffered from chronic pain, further influenced people's capacity to maintain hope and faith that G-d would get them through difficult times.

Then came the traumatic assassination of our visionary president, followed by the continuing television newscasts of our nation torn by conflict over the war in Vietnam. This was a period of grief and anger intermixed with a renewed sense of hope from changes in civil rights and from the inspirational leadership of such people as Martin Luther King, Jr. and Robert F. Kennedy. An array of poetic lyrics and songs written by various artists depicted how the times were definitely "a-changing." Many pain sufferers, once again, renewed their faith.

But faith in G-d and in those leaders in authority, let alone faith in any form of institution, spiraled downward as we experienced the assassinations of King and Kennedy, followed by Watergate and then religious sex abuse scandals. It's no wonder that many people turned from faith to anesthetizing substances to alleviate pain.

Now we have an addiction crisis.

Several years ago, I attended a Harvard University-sponsored conference on addictions where a reputable professor and researcher from my undergraduate alma mater, New York University, discussed the results of his studies on the reasons for Alcoholics Anonymous (AA) attendance. He identified, through statistical analysis, that the primary factor that influenced substance abusers to regularly attend thousands of daily AA meetings was, of all things, their need for spirituality and a belief in a higher power.

How ironic!

Have AA, Narcotics Anonymous, and Overeaters Anonymous replaced church, synagogue and mosque attendance?

Perhaps. Perhaps not.

At the end of each Saturday at synagogue service, we conclude with this verse: *"Do not fear sudden terror, nor the destruction of the wicked when it comes (Proverbs 3:23). Contrive a scheme, but it will be foiled; conspire a plot, but it will not materialize, for G-d is with you (Isaiah 2:10). To your old age, I am with you; I have made you and I will carry you. I will sustain you and deliver you"* (ibid. 46:4).

There is much comfort in this verse. The hope is that you should find comfort in any statements or acts of faith, especially if you experience chronic pain.

You are the navigator on your life jet! As the navigator, who can regulate all the dials (chronic pain rating scales), you must inevitably have ultimate faith that, no matter how much unexpected turbulence you experience, the Pilot will see you through it. Your faith in the Pilot is based on how much total control you believe you have in your life; consequently, your rating on spirituality is related to your control scale rating. There will be times when you feel helpless and powerless. If you can accept helplessness as part of the human condition, then you can have a high spirituality rating, whether that's faith in G-d or some higher power.

Read any books, short stories, quotations, poems, essays, or speeches that enhance your spirituality ratings.

Set aside some time each day as "sacred time," a term coined by Emile Durkheim. This could be religious attendance at a service, some spiritual period of study or simply a retreat for yourself to find a space away from stress, even for an hour, where you can meditate, reflect on aspects of your life that bring you meaningfulness, or simply de-stress.

Do something nice for somebody else! Doing good deeds will make you feel good and bring you meaning.

Read and memorize any specific spiritual verses that bring you reassurance that you are not alone. For some, these may be the sayings of Hillel, the psalms of King David, or Rabbi Nachman of Breslov. For others, it may be the teachings of Jesus, Mohammad, Confucius or Buddha. Choose those verses that bring you comfort.

Hillel, Ethics of the Fathers, 1:14:
"If I am only for myself, who am I? If not now, when?"

Psalm 130:
"Grant complete healing to all my wounds, for You, Almighty G-d, are a faithful and merciful healer."

Psalm 95:
"When I thought that my foot was slipping, Your kindness, O Lord, supported me. When my worrisome thoughts multiply within me, Your consolation delights my soul."

Psalm 86:
" Your kindness to me has been great; You have saved my soul from the depths of despair."

Psalm 25:
"Turn to me and be gracious to me, for I am alone and afflicted. The sufferings of my heart have increased; deliver me from my tribulations. Guard my soul and deliver me."

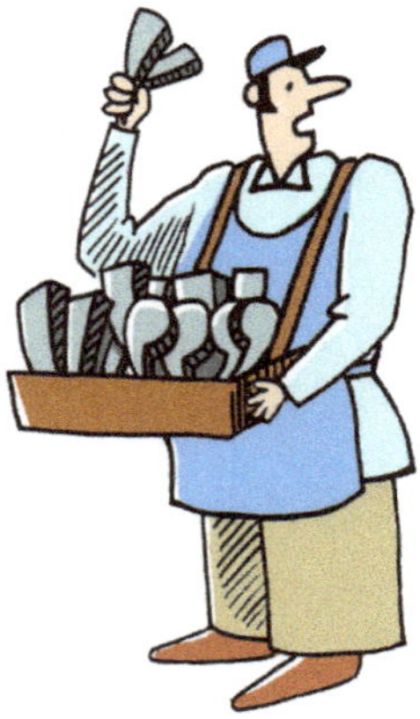

Get your red-hot motivational quotes here!

Isaiah:
" Answer me, O Lord, answer me for I am in great distress. Be near to my cry; let Your loving kindness console me."

Psalm 147:
"He heals the broken hearted and binds their wounds."

Psalm 31:
"Just knowing You are listening will quickly rescue me. For You are my boulder and fortress. Take me from this hidden snare, for You are my strength. The snare is the web of worry that my mind hides within me. It appears when I find myself trapped by doubt and fear. Hear my voice clearly saying, "You are my stronghold!" You see my suffering. You know the troubles of my soul. True joy comes from deep within my heart. For when I give myself over to You, I can actualize a sense of real exaltation."

Psalm 25:

"Our hearts become free of dread. No other person can see the extent of my personal suffering for it is unique to my own mind. Only You know what nibbles away at my soul. Have compassion on me, for I am in distress. My eyes, soul and innards waste away from anger and pain."

Psalm 23:

"The Lord is my shepherd: I shall not want. He maketh me to lie down in green pastures; He leadeth me beside the still waters; He restoreth my soul."

Luke 6:8,

"Do to others as you would have them do to you."

John 4:7,

"Let us love one another, for love comes from G-d. Everyone who loves has been born of G-d and knows G-d."

John 4:8,

"Whoever does not love does not know God, because God is love."

Prophet Mohammad:

"Those who love will be loved by the Most Loving. So love those on Earth and those in Heaven will love you."

Quran 25:63:

"The servants of the most loving are those who walk on the earth in humility, and when the ignorant address them, they say, 'Peace!' "

Quran 49:13:

"In G-d's eyes the most noble of you are those who are the most mindful of Him: G-d is all knowing, all aware."

Confucius:

"Wheresoever you go, go with all your heart!"

"What you do not want done to yourself, do not do to others."

"Wherever you go, there you are."

Buddha:

"You can search throughout the entire universe for someone who is more deserving of your love and affection than you are yourself, and that person is not to be found anywhere. You, yourself, as much as anybody in the entire universe, deserve your love and affection."

"When you realize how perfect everything is you will tilt your head back and laugh at the sky."

"I understand with love comes pain, but why did I have to love so much?"

Rabbi Nachman of Breslov:

"If you won't be better
tomorrow than you were today,
then what do you need tomorrow for?"

"Grant me the ability to be alone.
May it be my custom to go outdoors
each day among the trees and grasses
among all growing things and there may
I be alone, and enter into prayer to
talk with the one that I belong to."

"Get into the habit of singing
a tune. It will give you new life
and fill you with joy. Get into the
habit of (imagining yourself) dancing.
It will displace depression
and dispel hardship."

"Always wear a smile. The gift of life
will then be yours to give."

"While praying (Meditating), listen to
the words very carefully. When your
heart is attentive, your entire being
enters your prayer (Meditation)
without your having to force it."

"Prayers (Meditations)
truly from the heart open all
doors in Heaven."

"Find a day for yourself
-- better yet, late at night.
Go to the forest or to the field,
or lock yourself in a room ...
You will meet solitude there.
There you will be able to listen
attentively to the noise of the
wind first, to birds singing, to
see wonderful nature and to notice
yourself in it ... and to come
back to harmonic connection with
the world and its Creator."

"Just as your hand, held
before the eye, can hide the
tallest mountain, so this small
earthly life keeps us from seeing
the vast radiance that fills the
core of the universe."

"Even if you can't sing well,
sing. Sing to yourself. Sing in
the privacy of your home. But sing."

"The whole world
is a very narrow bridge.
And the most important thing
is not to be afraid."

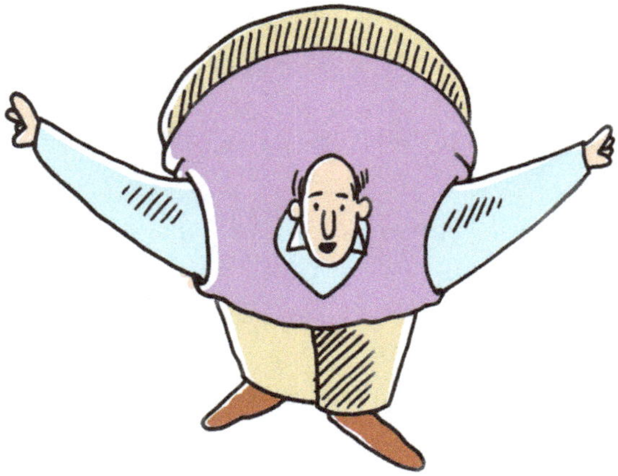

Take a bow for a pain less life!

Chapter 12: Conclusion

It should be clear by now that no one is free of pain, even from an early age. Don't let anyone tell you differently. Pain is a metaphor. It's not just your physical pain. If you thought that our opiate addiction crisis is bad, a recent study indicated a 50% increase in alcohol use disorders between 2012 and 2013. The largest increase is for people over 65. People are experiencing intense pain from experiences like obesity, diabetes, high cholesterol, lack of exercise, life stress, anxiety, depression, trauma, boredom, phone and other addictions, the need for immediate gratification, and a need to strengthen their fortitude skills. We have a significant "passive suicidal" crisis going on comparable to the Black Death Plague of the Middle Ages!

How you can reduce your chronic pain?

Perceive your chronic pain as a challenge, as an opportunity, rather than an experience of despair. You have the ability to fight it, and this book's model of a Pain Management Lifestyle gives you the tools to fight and triumph.

Acknowledgements

I wish to thank Aaron Beck and Martin Seligman for helping to transform our way of thinking and improving our health and happiness.

I wish to thank Kate Victory Hannisian of Blue Pencil Consulting for her diligence in proofreading and editing this book, and Brian Murphy of Brian Murphy Art and Design for his creative gift in graphic art and design.

I wish to thank my dear friend Roy Turnage, for his inspiration and for his allowing me to write on his scenic lake float with our beautiful dogs, Rudy and Dora.

Finally, I am forever grateful to my beautiful wife Stephanie, to whom I've been married for over forty years. My wife has experienced my ups and downs, my capacity to cope and be resilient and then lose it as I had such difficulty grieving who I once was as an invigorated athlete. Stephanie is a natural optimist, being this way even in childhood as an oldest, responsible sibling. Over time, she has earned the respect and loyalty of her colleagues and friends as a leader in psychiatric social work and administration. She has a keen sense of empathic intuition that certainly came in handy, especially when knowing my tolerance was low and I became a bear to live with. Whenever I generated catastrophic thoughts, Stephanie had that natural ability to turn defeatism into optimism, being the cheerleader once again as she was for her high school back in the early 1970s. She is a beautiful human being and I have been so fortunate to have had her as my main coach during my ordeal.

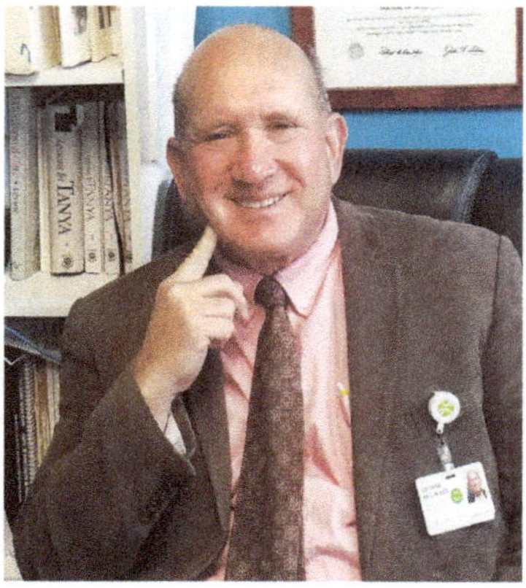

About the Author

George Beilin, EdD, is a seasoned, licensed psychologist with over 50 years of clinical experience and has specialized in the treatment of patients who have chronic pain. He obtained his master's degree in 1972 and his doctorate in psychology in 1976 from Boston University. Dr. Beilin was the chief psychologist for the pain center at Lahey Outpatient Center at Danvers, Massachusetts, where he evaluated and treated multiple patients for various pain disorders. He has facilitated a free, weekly chronic pain support group.

Dr. Beilin formulated his theoretical model for reducing chronic pain from his interest in the trans-theoretical model of change and a bio-psycho-social approach to perceiving pain as being influenced by multiple sources other than simply physical ones. He emphasizes building fortitude to re-frame chronic pain as a challenge rather than an obstruction in one's life. His empathy for patients with chronic pain stems from enduring his own chronic pain from six major surgeries in seven years.

Dr. Beilin has been married for over 40 years to his wife, Stephanie, a Licensed Psychiatric Social Worker who is employed by the Danvers Public Schools. They reside in Hamilton, Massachusetts.